Natural Pregnancy, Natural Baby

Natural Pregnancy, Natural Baby

Natural Remedies for Pregnancy, Birth and Post-Partum Discomforts

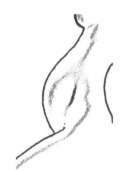

Dr. Stacey Rosenberg
Chiropractor
DipGS, BAppSci(Clinical)/BChiroSci, DC

www.GibsonsChiropractic.com
chiropractor@dccnet.com

To order additional copies of this book, contact:
Xlibris Corporation
1-888-795-4274
www.Xlibris.com
Orders@Xlibris.com
36960

Contents

Acknowledgements

This book really came about as a result of my two beautiful pregnancies. My wonderful midwives and our local Bellies and Babies Support Network provided me with so much useful information in the form of handouts that I got inspired to put it all together for them! At first I thought it would only be a couple pages put together as a handout on herbs to use in pregnancy but it just kept growing and growing and GROWING! After I put together the information on herbs, I then realized there wasn't much out there on homeopathic remedies and that I should add the information I had gleaned from a workshop provided by a local classical homeopath and former midwife. And then I thought, "Gee, what about your 'real' area of expertise?" I hadn't even included much information on chiropractic, which can be a huge help during pregnancy. So that *had* to be in the book! And then other ideas, such as more information on pre-natal yoga and natural treatments for infant conditions came to mind until I finally had to say, "Whoa! Enough already! You'll never finish this if you don't stop there!"

So I really have many people to thank for helping me put this all together. First of all, I have to thank my husband Udo and my daughter Saĵa for being so patient with me while I plugged away on the computer for what I'm sure seemed like endless hours during the hot summer months. I should also thank my son Jäger as he had to put up with Mommy sitting for hours typing while he was in utero (and for allowing me the energy and providing the motivation to take this project on while pregnant). I really have to thank my two lovely midwives Anne Marie (Aus) and Petra for a lot of the handouts that formed the initial information and starting point for further research and for inspiring and encouraging me to finish this book. (And for also proofreading the first draft!) And I need to thank my Aunty Karen, Sheryl, Berni, Kim, Penny and especially Angela for proofreading, providing helpful suggestions and improvements, and encouragement. And I need to thank Oryane Belair, Marlee Berman, Dr. Karen Bagnell, Dr. Jeanne Ohm, Janice Clarfield, Dr. Don Nixdorf and several others for providing some of the information and articles (and advice) that I used as well. And last but certainly not least, thank you to my Mom and Grandmother for their encouragement over the years and for picking most of the herbs that I photographed and scanned.

I really hope this book will help expectant mothers feel more empowered to use natural remedies the way that I did to help relieve some of the common complaints we all experience while pregnant. I also hope this book will help inform some of the pregnancy care providers as to what's out there—natural and safe—to use to help ease those complaints. After all, it's not just about providing mom with relief but ultimately it's about giving baby the best chance to have a happy and healthy start to life!

1

Introduction

Congratulations! You're going to have a baby!

Now as you take off on your journey towards parenthood, there is much planning and learning to take place! Being pregnant is a momentous time in a woman's life and preparing for a new baby is a daunting challenge for even the most organized mothers-to-be. Becoming a parent is an exciting life experience, especially if you are expecting your first child. During the pregnancy, as your baby and belly grows, you are filled with wishes, hopes and dreams. Your thoughts are filled with promise and your emotions are heightened. Learning that you are soon to become a parent can produce many emotions—from happiness, surprise and anticipation to anxiety and concern about what lies in store. Such feelings are natural, for pregnancy and the so-called fourth trimester (post-partum period) of caring for a new baby is often a time of great change. Knowing what to expect can make the coming changes easier to handle and enjoy.

Sure, there are discomforts, especially in the summer when the heat can get to you! But despite the aches and pains that come with pregnancy, carrying a baby to term is an incredible experience. Symptoms and discomfort can arise from the natural changes in your body: hormonal fluctuations, breast enlargement in preparation for lactation, increased respiration, increased blood flow, increased demand on the kidneys, softening of the pelvic joints, as well as increased sensitivity to foods and smells. Most of these changes can be managed by natural adjustments to foods and lifestyle. And it would be surprising if you weren't tired—in some ways, your pregnant body is working harder even when you're resting than a non-pregnant body is when mountain-climbing—you just can't see its efforts! Symptoms of imbalance are messages to take better care of yourself—dietary changes, use of herbs or homeopathy, consulting a chiropractor, or other natural remedies can help bring you back into balance. This book is intended to help you work to prevent and treat common pregnancy, birth and post-partum complaints before they affect you or your peace of mind!

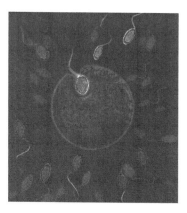

From the moment of conception, your body goes through a series of remarkable changes. There are millions of different hormonal changes and chemical reactions occurring both in the mother and the developing baby—all of which are controlled and coordinated through the nervous system. Now more than ever, you need a nervous system that responds immediately and accurately to changing requirements in all parts of your body; therefore you need a healthy spine.

New cells are created to form the two and a half extra pounds of uterine muscle, two pounds of amniotic fluid, placenta (about one pound), a fifty per cent increase in blood volume (approximately four pounds), an extra three pounds in the breasts, about five to eight pounds of extra body stores for pregnancy and breastfeeding as well as the brain, nerves, muscles, tissues, organs, and skin of your baby. Additionally, you will need to replace many more of your own kidney and liver cells that are used to process the waste of two rather than one. You and your child are formed from and maintained by the nourishment you receive in the forty weeks of pregnancy so it is *vital* that you ensure you are eating well and getting adequate amounts of the essential nutrients that are needed to sustain a healthy pregnancy—for both you and the baby!

Summary of Your Baby's Growth In Utero

Week	Month	Your Baby's Growth	Weight (Averages)	Length
1 2 3	1	Baby is conceived and begins developing.	-	1/5 in. 1 mm.
4 5 6 7 8	2	Baby's heart begins beating; and its brain, spinal cord, arms, legs, eyes, nose and mouth begin developing.	-	2 in. 5 cm.
9 10 11 12	3	Baby's eyes are closed and fingernails are developing. Testes and ovaries have formed.	⅓ oz./10 gr. ½ oz./15 gr.	3 in. 7.5 cm
13 14 15 16	4	Baby's legs are well developed. Breathing and swallowing motions begin.	2oz./60 gr. 4oz./120 gr.	6 in. 15 cm.
17 18 19 20	5	Baby's hands can grasp and it can hiccup. Toenails are developing. Mother can now feel baby's movement.	7oz./210 gr. 11⅓ oz./340 gr.	10 in. 25 cm
21 22 23 24	6	Baby can make a fist and hair is visible. Its skin is thin, red and wrinkled.	1lb. 2oz./540 gr. 1 lb. 6 oz./660 gr.	12 in. 30 cm.
25 26 27 28 29	7	Baby has eyelashes and its body is thin. Baby can hear sounds, especially mother's voice.	1lb. 13oz./870 gr. 2lbs. 3oz./1.05 kg. 2lbs.	13.8 in. 34.5 cm 14.4 in. 36 cm 15 in.
30 31 32	8	Baby can open its eyes and is practising to breathe.	14oz./1.38 kg. 3lbs. 12oz./1.8 kg. 4lbs.	37.5 cm 16.5 in. 41.25 cm 17.7 in.
33 34 35 36	9	Baby responds to familiar voices and is gaining four to eight ounces (115 to 230 grams) a week.	10oz./2.22 kg. 5lbs. 8oz./2.64 kg.	44.25 cm 18.3 in. 45.75 cm
37 38 39	10	Baby is growing and gaining weight. Baby is now ready to be born!	6lbs. 6oz./3.06 kg 7lbs. 8oz./3.6 kg.	18.9 in. 47.25 cm. 19.6 in. 49 cm.

Every pregnant woman experiences some kind of discomfort during her pregnancy. But pregnancy is a special time to reflect on your family's plans and dreams—not a time to struggle with discomfort or pain. You are all-important to your developing unborn child. You are your infant's universe—the ultimate provider. What an awesome responsibility! Most women know this intuitively, and medical science is building clinical evidence that confirms how important you are. Strive to give your baby the gift of a calm, comfortable and natural pregnancy and birth—how we come into the world influences the rest of our life! During this meaningful time, be proactive and endeavour to prevent common pregnancy and birth-related discomforts before they distract you from focusing on your family's health, happiness, harmony and well being. If you're a first-time expectant mother, enjoy what will probably be your last chance for a long while to focus on taking care of yourself without feeling guilty!

Every pregnancy should be a wanted pregnancy and every child should be a wanted child. Pre-natal bonding can help you work to create a loving, joyous, nurturing pregnancy and birth experience for yourself and your baby.

Mother's Conversation with Her Unborn Child

When you're born, little baby, I will give you love so that you grow in love and trust yourself and others.
I promise to talk to you in a way that you will listen, and I promise to listen to you in such a way that you will talk.
I will respect your right to be yourself, and I'll try to help you to learn to respect the rights of others.
I promise to encourage you to seek answers that will lead you to know and appreciate this wonderful world around you.
I promise to teach you with love and guidance, rather than anger and punishment.
I will teach you and I will learn from you.
I will provide opportunities for you to help you grow in love and happiness.
I see you, little baby, coming from my womb; and I see you cradled in my arms.
I'm elated at the thought of your coming from me.
Dear Little Baby, I Love You.[1]

---

[1] Reprinted with permission from the Hypnobirthing® Institute—www.Hypno-Birthing.com.

Since the ear is one of the earliest organs to fully develop, the sense of hearing is perhaps our most direct and reliable connection to the baby. In his book, "The Secret Life of the Unborn Child," Dr. Thomas Verny writes, "Recent studies show that from the twenty-fourth week on, the unborn child listens all the time." Given this, what would be the most important sounds to have in baby's environment? By far, his parents' voices are top choice. Next is music. While everyone has his or her own personal musical preferences, the choice of which music to play for the baby is very clear. In an arresting series of new studies, it has been shown that the unborn child has distinct musical likes and dislikes—and discriminating ones at that. Vivaldi is one of the unborn child's favourite composers; Mozart is another. Whenever one of their soaring compositions was put on, foetal heart rates invariably steadied and kicking declined. The music of Brahms and Beethoven and all kinds of rock, on the other hand, drove most foetuses to distraction. They kicked violently when records of these composers were played to their pregnant mothers.

Repeated exposure to the same song and to its mother's voice has notable benefits to the child, and another beneficiary is the mom-to-be. This time of relaxation and focus on the coming of the baby produces calming chemicals in the blood that are transferred to the baby through the placenta. These chemicals allow baby and mother to share the bonding experience, laying a foundation for later learning. Parents should communicate with their children as often as possible, even while they are still in utero. A wonderful example of a book to read to your unborn child is "Oh, Baby, the Places You'll Go!" by Tish Rabe which uses the Dr. Seuss pattern of rhythm and rhyme. When mother sings or reads to her baby, the familiar sound of her voice has a calming, comforting effect. It is also a wonderful opportunity to start establishing a routine, even before your baby is born, which will become increasingly important after your baby is born as he/she continues to grow and develop. Your baby needs to feel close and secure with you. Hearing their mother's (and father's) voice provides familiarity and continuity with the person they have been with since before their birth. Babies keenly want to connect with their parents—always feeling safe, loved and looked after. It is also during these moments that children are most receptive to learning. Additionally, studies have shown that how often children are spoken and read to is a significant predictor of future reading skills and success in school. So sing, talk, and read to, and later, with your baby—it's never too early to start!

Preparing to welcome a baby is a life-changing experience. This book hopes to offer techniques, exercises, nutritional advice and natural remedies to help ease you through pregnancy, birth and the post-partum period. This book is designed to serve the ninety-five per cent of families whose pregnancies fall into the normal, low or no risk categories. The content of this book is not intended to replace the advice and/or care of a health-care provider. It is not intended to be an exhaustive, stage-by-stage pregnancy manual either. If you need a resource that is technical and medically-descriptive in nature, please see the *References and Resources* section at the end of this book. It is intended to assist in this transition into parenthood and becoming a family and to supplement some of the excellent resources already out there. You should always seek the advice of a qualified, professional caregiver for all pregnancy-related matters.

2

Natural Pregnancy and Birth

Natural pregnancy and birth is very simply having a baby without using drugs.

A common phrase heard when talking with people about natural birthing practices is, "birth is a natural process, not a medical procedure." In today's society, this is definitely a radical concept for most doctors, but it is true nonetheless. You really can have a beautiful, drug-free experience even if you have your baby in a hospital. You simply need to know it is possible, you need to find a doctor or midwife who will support you in your point of view, and you need to prepare yourself so you can relax and let nature take its course.

Natural childbirth is based on the premise that pregnancy and childbirth are normal physiological processes that, in most cases, can be expected to occur normally. Women should see themselves as inherently healthy and want to experience their pregnancy, labour and birth from that perspective and to be in charge of their own bodies and experience. Promoting health and well being throughout the pregnancy and birth is key, while maintaining a focus on preventing complications, early identification of potential problems and appropriate intervention.

The advantages of a natural childbirth are huge. Three big advantages are:

1. Natural childbirth is much better for the mother. You have a completely different experience during birth if you are not drugged—a significantly more fulfilling and beautiful experience. The confidence in your strength and capabilities that you can gain are, perhaps, the ideal preparation for meeting the challenges of parenting. You also feel much more in control of your body and the health of your baby.

2. Natural childbirth is much better for the baby. The baby arrives in an undrugged and much more active and alert state. It is amazing to see videotapes showing the differences between drugged and undrugged babies immediately after birth. Undrugged babies are active and responsive. Drugged babies can barely move.

3. Natural childbirth is much better for the family. When an alert and active (undrugged) baby is placed on the abdomen of an alert and undrugged mother, an amazing thing happens: the baby and mother bond in a significant and real way. The baby will naturally find the breast and begin feeding. The baby will make significant eye contact with the mother and father and respond to them. This simply does not happen when mother and child are drugged, and as a result breastfeeding starts off on a much rockier road.

What most people don't realize is that any drug given to a woman in labour will reach her baby in less than five minutes, and in an adult dose. If the chemicals are strong enough to help relieve pain in an adult, they can certainly affect a newborn. These very powerful narcotics and analgesics can lower maternal hormone levels and slow down labour, causing serious problems in the newborn, such as respiratory distress, sucking problems, unresponsiveness and inability to bond, sometimes lasting for weeks. Labour drugs cross the blood/brain and placental barriers, and will be transported into the breast milk as well. Epidurals can contain opiate painkillers just like narcotics, can prolong second stage of labour, can lead to assisted birth practices such as forceps or vacuum extraction, can lower the mother's blood pressure, sometimes dangerously so, and the baby then can suffer foetal distress. The mother can also experience negative effects from the epidural, such as incomplete relief, no relief at all, chronic back problems, spinal headache, allergic reaction, itching, breathing difficulties, painful and/or difficult breastfeeding, and other serious adverse effects.

The use of drugs during pregnancy, labour and delivery contain a special risk since they affect two people—you and the baby. As all drugs (and even some herbs) have some risk, the risk and the benefit must be weighed. At appropriate times and after careful consideration, drugs can and do save lives. However, properly prepared pregnant couples *rarely* need drugs for the birth of their baby. It is better to have an unmedicated pregnancy and birth, in most cases, for the mother and her baby. You can achieve the goal of an easier, more comfortable, and safer birth, without unnecessary medication!

Make no mistake about it—you cannot have a natural pregnancy and childbirth in today's society unless you take active steps to make it happen. You and your spouse must decide in your own minds that you want a natural pregnancy and birth. You must find a doctor or midwife who supports that decision (see *Questions to Ask Your Pregnancy Health Care Provider*). The focus of visits with your chosen caregiver should be about promoting a healthy pregnancy, labour, birth, and baby, while educating and enabling you to actively participate in the decision-making. You and your spouse must train for the birth so you know what to expect, how to manage discomfort and what to do at different stages of the birth. You also need to prepare a birth plan so that you can state your desires about a host of variables including: drugs, foetal monitoring, episiotomies, IVs, birth positions, etc. (see *Sample Birth Plan*). The number of options can be bewildering but it is amazing how all of these options actually make sense once you have done the research into the type of pregnancy and birth you want. You don't have to use drugs, and you don't have to suffer either, while giving your baby life. You *can* enjoy your natural pregnancy and baby's birth!

[Adapted from: http://www.bygpub.com/natural/natural-childbirth.htm]

3

Questions to Ask Your Pregnancy Health Care Provider

These are some of the questions you may wish to ask when interviewing your potential health care provider.

The answers should help you decide if you are comfortable entrusting your baby's birth to this particular practitioner—and always remember that if you are not comfortable with the answers and the practitioner is unwilling to accommodate your wishes, it is your *right* to change providers at *any* time. Your caregiver should practice and facilitate informed choice as well as actively promote and support your decision-making throughout the pregnancy, birth, and post-partum care.

1. How long have you been practising? How many births have you attended?
2. What percentage of the births were c-sections?
3. Do you attend home births?
4. What's your standard schedule or frequency of pre-natal appointments?
5. How much time do you set aside for each pre-natal visit?
6. What types of tests are you likely to recommend over the course of my pregnancy?
7. What percentage of your patients write birth plans? What advice would you offer if I decide to write one?
8. Under what circumstances, if any, would you transfer my care to another healthcare provider (e.g. a specialist)?

9. Under what circumstances do you induce labour?
10. How much time will you be able to spend with me while I'm in labour?
11. Do the majority of your patients choose medicated or unmedicated/ natural births?
12. What methods of pharmacological and non-pharmacological pain relief (e.g. comfort measures) do you recommend most often?
13. Do you encourage couples to attempt unmedicated deliveries?
14. How do you feel if I were to decide to use the services of a doula or other labour support person?
15. How do you feel about using natural or alternative therapies such as chiropractic, herbs and homeopathy during pregnancy and labour?
16. Do you routinely use electronic foetal monitoring during labour?
17. Do you routinely use IV's during labour?
18. What percentage of women in your care receive episiotomies?
19. Will my baby be able to remain with me after the birth (e.g. rooming in)?
20. Do you provide breastfeeding support?
21. Do you routinely use antibiotic ointment in the baby's eyes immediately after delivery?
22. Do you routinely do vitamin K injections in the baby?
23. What types of neo-natal testing to you normally do?
24. What are your feelings on vaccinations?
25. How often will I see you in the post-partum period? Should or will my baby be checked by another health care provider during this period?
26. How do I contact you in an emergency and what times are you unavailable (e.g. are you taking any holidays)? Who should I call instead?

4

Sample Birth Plan

Birth Plan for: _____

Due Date:
Patient of:
Scheduled to deliver at:
Husband/Partner/Caretaker:

To whom it may concern:

Following is a statement of my birth plan and childbirth choices. I have educated myself prior to making these decisions and hope to carry them out, but I realize that complications do arise and in such instances trust my caretaker(s) _____ to make necessary decisions on my behalf.

I look forward to sharing my upcoming birth with you. I have created the following birth plan to help you understand my preferences for my upcoming labour and delivery. I fully understand that in certain circumstances these guidelines may not be followed, but it is my hope that you will assist me in making this the experience I hope for. Thank you for taking the time to read this and helping me realize my birth plan. I thank you in advance for your support and kind attention to our choices. We know you join us in looking forward to a beautiful birth. If you have any questions or suggestions, please let me know.

Sincerely,

Date: _____

Labour

- I will be staying at home as long as possible during labour.
- I would like to be able to return home until labour progresses further if less than 4 centimetres dilated and other factors do not warrant admission.
- I would like to be free to walk around during labour.
- I wish to be able to move around and change position at will throughout labour.
- I would like to be able to have fluids by mouth throughout labour.
- I prefer no restrictions on eating or drinking.
- I will be bringing my own music to play during labour.
- I would like the environment to be kept as quiet as possible.
- I would like the lights in the room to be kept low during my labour.
- I would prefer to keep the number of vaginal exams to a minimum.
- I do not want an IV unless I become dehydrated.
- I do not want IV or oral antibiotics, even if the membranes have been ruptured more than twenty-four hours, unless clinically indicated (e.g. positive Streptococcus B culture)
- I would like to wear contact lenses or glasses at all times when conscious.
- I would prefer to avoid an enema and/or shaving of pubic hair.

Monitoring

- I do not wish to have continuous foetal monitoring unless it is required by the condition of my son/daughter.
- I do not want an internal monitor unless my son/daughter has shown some sign of distress.
- I prefer Doppler for monitoring.

Labour Augmentation/Induction

- To consider inducement only if onset of labour is unusually delayed and if there is medical urgency.
- To use only natural means of inducement, moving to prostaglandin gel, Pitocin drip or other procedures as a last resort.
- I would prefer to be allowed to try changing position and other natural methods (walking, nipple stimulation) before Pitocin is administered, and to be accorded the uninterrupted privacy to do so.
- I prefer to utilize homeopathy, acupressure, prostaglandin gel or stripping the membranes if augmentation is necessary.
- I do not wish to have the amniotic membrane ruptured artificially unless signs of foetal distress require internal monitoring.

Anaesthesia/Pain Medication

- I decline discussion on pain tolerance and pain levels.
- I ask that staff honour our need for quiet and refrain from references to "pain", "hurt", or to offer medication unless requested.
- I realize that many pain medications exist—I'll ask for them if I need them.
- I plan to deliver without pain medication and will be using Hypnobirthing®, water (tub/shower), heat/cold, massage, chiropractic, acupressure, homeopathy, and birth breathing to cope.

Caesarean

- Unless absolutely necessary, I would like to avoid a caesarean.
- If a caesarean delivery is indicated, I would like to be fully informed and to participate in the decision-making process.
- I would like my husband/partner present at all times if my son/daughter requires a caesarean delivery.
- If my son/daughter is not in distress, my son/daughter should be given *immediately* to _____ after the delivery.

Episiotomy

- I would prefer not to have an episiotomy unless absolutely required for the baby's safety.
- I am hoping to protect the perineum. I am practicing ahead of time by squatting, doing Kegel exercises, and perineal massage.
- I will be using birth breathing primarily instead of pushing, to gently nudge the baby down the birth path.
- I prefer to tear than episiotomy and I would like a local anaesthetic to repair a tear or an episiotomy.

Delivery

- I would prefer to birth in an atmosphere of gentle encouragement during the final birthing phase without "coaching." Please—calm, low tones, free of "pushing" prompts.
- I would like to use mother-directed breathing to facilitate the descent of the baby, as much as possible, until crowning takes place.
- I would appreciate guidance in when to breathe/push and when to stop so the perineum can stretch.
- I would like to be allowed to choose the position in which I give birth, including squatting.
- I would like my husband/partner and/or nurses to support me and my legs as necessary during the pushing stage.

- I would like to try to deliver in a hands-and-knees position.
- I would like to try to deliver in a squatting position, using my husband/partner, a birthing stool, ball or a squatting bar for support.
- I would like to remain in the tub or shower for as long as possible.
- I prefer that no forceps or vacuum extraction be used except in *extreme* circumstances.
- I would like a mirror available so I can see my son/daughter's head when it crowns.
- I would like the chance to touch my son/daughter's head when it crowns.
- I would appreciate having the room lights turned low for the actual delivery.
- I would appreciate having the room as quiet as possible when my son/daughter is born.
- I would like to have my son/daughter placed on my stomach/chest immediately after delivery.

Immediately After Delivery

- I would prefer that the umbilical cord stop pulsating before it is cut.
- I would like to have my husband/partner and caretaker _____ _____ to cut the cord.
- I would prefer that the birth is complete before using any suctioning on the baby.
- I would prefer that the vernix be absorbed into the baby's skin; delay cleaning or rubbing and to use a soft cloth when rubbing is appropriate.
- I would like to hold my son/daughter, if possible, while I deliver the placenta and any tissue repairs are made.
- I would like to have my son/daughter evaluated and bathed in my presence.
- I plan to keep my son/daughter near me following birth and would appreciate if the evaluation of my son/daughter can be done with my son/daughter on my abdomen, with both of us covered by a warm blanket, unless there is an unusual situation.
- I would prefer to hold my son/daughter rather than have him/her placed under heat lamps.
- I would prefer no cord traction, Pitocin or manual removal of the placenta unless there is an emergency.
- I would prefer to allow up to thirty minutes if necessary for natural placenta expulsion with use of immediate breast feeding, uterine massage and/or nipple stimulation to assist the birth of the placenta.

- After the birth, I would prefer to be given a few moments of privacy to urinate on my own before being catheterized.
- If my son/daughter must be taken from me to receive medical treatment, my husband or some other person I designate will accompany my son/daughter at all times.
- If my son/daughter is transported to another facility, move us as soon as possible.
- I would like to delay the eye medication for my son/daughter until at least couple hours after birth, and only to be used if clinically indicated (*not* routine administration).
- I wish to delay vitamin K injection: to be used only if delivery is prolonged, traumatic or otherwise clinically indicated. I would prefer that oral vitamin K supplements to be used if available.

Postpartum
- I would like a private room.
- Unless required for health reasons, I do not wish to be separated from my son/daughter.
- I would like to have 'room in' and my son/daughter to be with me at all times, though I will be going home with my son/daughter as soon as possible.
- I would like to delay PKU, CH, GS, and MCAD and any other routine blood tests for my son/daughter until day three after the delivery.

Breastfeeding
- I plan to breastfeed my son/daughter and would like to begin nursing very shortly after birth.
- I plan to breastfeed several times in the first few hours after the birth.
- Unless medically necessary, I do not wish to have any bottles given to my son/daughter (including glucose water or plain water).
- I do not want my son/daughter to be given a pacifier.

Circumcision
- I do/do not want my son circumcised.

Photo/Video
- Photographs to be taken only of labour, and after the birth (not of the delivery).

Other
- I would prefer that no students, interns, residents or non-essential personnel be present during my labour or the birth—only necessary hospital staff or cheerful observers, please.

- There is the possibility that relatives other than my husband and daughter, and _____ may make *brief* visits during labour and after the birth.
- I would prefer/prefer not to have telephone inquiries relayed to my room.

[Adapted from: http://www.birthplan.com].

5

Fifty Comfort Measures to Ease Labour Pain

Comfort measures are strategies designed to help you cope with the discomfort of labour.

A good childbirth preparation class should teach you an assortment of ways to cope, as will many books.

Benefits of Using Comfort Measures

Basically, there are three ways of handling labour discomfort: comfort measures, narcotics (opiates) and regional analgesia, which consists of epidurals, intrathecal or spinal injections, and their combinations. Comfort measures are about as effective as narcotics at making labour tolerable. However, narcotics can potentially have adverse effects on you and your baby. And regional analgesia, while offering superior pain relief, can cause a host of problems not only for you and your baby, but for the labour as well.

Comfort measures:

- Do not inhibit labour and in many cases, can enhance labour progress: mobility and activities like pelvic rocking help the baby shift into the optimal position for birth. Upright postures allow gravity to help the baby open the cervix and descend into the birth canal. Strategies to relax muscles keep muscle tension from impeding the work of the uterus. Cognitive techniques reduce fear and therefore associated tension. Emotional distress, as opposed to the healthy, normal stress of labour, can interfere with labour directly through the production of stress hormones and through the increased tension it causes. After all, the uterus is just like any other healthy muscle of the body and we don't expect flexing our biceps (arm) muscle within the normal range of motion will cause pain (until possibly the next day, if we've overdone it). Fear creates tension; tension creates pain and prevents the uterine muscles from working as effectively as they should. Fear and stress can also interfere with labour indirectly by preventing women from paying attention to their bodies and working effectively with their labours.

- Promote a sense of mastery: studies show that the key to a positive labour experience is the feeling that you have control over events and can cope with what is happening to you. Comfort measures make you the active agent in helping yourself. This is an important component for creating a sense of mastery.
- Facilitate endorphin production: during periods of intense physical demand and stress, the body produces natural painkillers called "endorphins." In a case of "no pain, no gain," endorphins are also responsible for the exhilaration and joy that can follow such periods.
- Enable you to postpone the use of pain medication: medications are more likely to cause problems with repeated doses, when different types of drugs are mixed, and with prolonged use. By using comfort measures, you may need only one dose of a narcotic instead of three, you may avoid using both a narcotic and an epidural, or you may delay having an epidural.
- Can instantly be stopped if it doesn't help or in the unlikely event that it causes trouble, for example, if the baby doesn't like you to be in some particular position, you can simply find another one. Pain medications, once administered, cannot be rescinded, and you may need another drug or procedure to remedy the ill effects. These, in turn, can introduce their own risks.

Potential Drawbacks of Using Comfort Measures

Comfort measures may not provide adequate relief of discomfort. This can lead to a feeling of personal failure if you wanted an unmedicated birth. Still, this will rarely be the case where caregivers and loved ones respect and support your desire to avoid pain medication, acknowledge your efforts to do so, and validate your disappointment at not achieving that goal.

How Comfort Measures Might Affect Your Birth Experience and Post-Partum Recovery

As with any experience that pushes you to your limits, an unmedicated labour can be a transformational event that changes how you think of yourself forever. Your pride in your achievement, the confidence in your strength and capabilities that you can gain are, perhaps, the ideal preparation for meeting the challenges of parenting. Avoiding or delaying the use of pain medication also gives you your best chance of having a complication-free labour and a healthy baby, which may mean an easier post-partum recovery.

Common Comfort Measures

- Environment:

  ◊ dim lights, candles
  ◊ peaceful surroundings
  ◊ privacy, warmth, music

- Physical:

  ◊ walking
  ◊ pelvic rocking
  ◊ using pillows for comfort
  ◊ standing, leaning, slow dancing with partner
  ◊ leaning or sitting on birth ball, swaying
  ◊ lying down (side-lying, semi-reclining, on the back, on the back with a tilt to the side)
  ◊ squatting, supported squatting
  ◊ leaping frog position
  ◊ lunging or kneeling on one knee
  ◊ hands and knees (with or without the birthing ball)
  ◊ lifting up the abdomen
  ◊ relaxation/tension release
  ◊ progressive tensing and then relaxation of body parts

- Touch:

  ◊ chiropractic adjustment
  ◊ massage (hand, foot, back)
  ◊ stroking

◊ cuddling, kissing
◊ counter-pressure against lower back
◊ double hip squeeze
◊ acupressure

- Heat:

  ◊ deep tub bath/whirlpool/hydrotherapy
  ◊ shower
  ◊ heated rice sock (or magic bag) on abdomen/groin or back
  ◊ hot packs to the perineum to help it relax and stretch

- Cold:

  ◊ ice packs on lower back
  ◊ cold packs to the perineum after the birth
  ◊ cool cloth to wipe face
  ◊ ice chips, popsicles or frozen fruit to suck/chew on
  ◊ open a window or fan your face and body

- Cognitive:

  ◊ visualization, guided imagery
  ◊ affirmations
  ◊ self-hypnosis
  ◊ focusing on the breath, birth breathing (e.g. visualizing filling a balloon with your breath)
  ◊ structured/patterned breathing patterns
  ◊ non-focused awareness (paying attention to everything you see, hear, feel, smell without focusing on any particular thing)
  ◊ counting off ten second intervals during contractions
  ◊ counting breaths
  ◊ chant, mantra, song, counting, prayer

- Aromatherapy

- Vocalizing: moaning and groaning

- Labour companion:

  ◊ the continuous presence of an experienced woman (e.g. a doula) can reduce the use of pain medication in general and of epidurals in particular. The presence of male partners, however desirable, doesn't seem to have this effect.

◊ feedback, verbal reminders, encouragement, reassurance, compliments, expressions of love

◊ undivided attention, immediate response to contractions, take charge routine, eye contact

6

Things You Should and Should Not Do During Pregnancy

There are quite a few things you can do during your pregnancy to help improve your and your baby's health.

You can also avoid risks that can complicate or terminate a pregnancy. For example, you probably know that getting enough folic acid is important. But did you know it is just as important to avoid cats? You probably knew that x-rays are harmful to the foetus, but did you know about electric blankets? Some of the items listed here are controversial. Some studies have shown they are dangerous, others not. It is up to you to do the research and decide if the risks outweigh the benefits.

Things You Should Do

Get Regular Medical and Chiropractic Exams

One of the easiest and best ways to avoid problems and complications during pregnancy is to get regular medical exams from your doctor or midwife. Also, get checked regularly by your family chiropractor to ensure that your pelvis is functioning correctly. "So long as the pelvis is in a balanced state, the ligaments connected to the uterus maintain an equalized, supportive suspension for the uterus. If your pelvis is out of balance in any way, these ligaments become torqued and twisted, causing a condition known as constraint to your uterus." (See *Chiropractic and Pregnancy: Greater Comfort and Safer Births* section).

Get the RDA (Recommended Daily Allowance) for Folic Acid

By getting the proper amount of folic acid you significantly reduce your baby's risk for spinal bifida. The current recommendation is 0.4 milligrams of folic acid daily (see *Folate/Folic Acid* section).

Take Pre-natal Vitamins

Both you and your baby need plenty of vitamins during pregnancy. Though it is better to get what you both need from diet, by taking special pre-natal vitamins you guarantee that you are not missing anything you need. Getting the proper vitamins can also help you avoid gestational diabetes (see *Basic Pregnancy Diet*).

Eat Plenty of Protein

The RDA of protein for pregnant women is seventy-five grams but one hundred grams is often recommended. Adequate protein is essential for the development of the baby (especially the brain) and may help protect against pre-eclampsia during pregnancy (see *Basic Pregnancy Diet*).

Eat Well and Get Plenty of Exercise.

Your diet needs to include plenty of vitamins, minerals, fibre and so on, just as it normally should. You also need to exercise and watch your weight as you normally would (see *Basic Pregnancy Diet* and *Pregnancy Exercise Tips* in the *An Expectant Parent's Guide to Chiropractic* sections).

Be Sure to Get Enough Fat in Your Diet

Fat and cholesterol, which you normally try to avoid, are important for absorbing the fat-soluble vitamins (A, D, E, and K) and for stretchable skin. Fat is also necessary for the developing baby's brain. That does not mean you want to be over-consuming it, but you need to make sure you are getting enough. There are so many fat-free foods on the market today (fat free milk, butter, ice cream, meat, bread, cookies, etc.), that it is very easy to consume a fat-free diet without realizing it. Two tablespoons of fat a day is recommended for pregnant women. Also, certain types of fat are more important as described in the Basic Pregnancy Diet.

Do Kegel Exercises

Weak Kegel muscles can contribute to pain during birth, premature flexion of the baby's head and a prolonged second stage. Childbirth can also weaken these muscles and cause discomfort afterwards (see the *Returning the Uterus, Perineum, and Abdominal Muscles to Normal More Quickly* or *An Expectant Parent's Guide to Chiropractic* sections for how to perform Kegel Exercises).

Use House Plants

A modern house is full of hundreds of hidden chemicals that are emitted by paints and stains, carpet, particle board, household cleaners and so on. One of the best ways to filter and remove these chemicals is with houseplants. Spider plants, for example, are known to be good at removing formaldehyde (which is quite common in paints). Also try using a HEPA filter air purifier.

Focus on Your Child and Avoid Negative Thoughts and Actions

Many books and articles discuss the importance of pre-natal bonding and the benefits of avoiding stress and negative thoughts (see the *References and Resources* section for more information).

Take Care When Traveling

Traveling when pregnant requires some special considerations, especially when traveling to foreign countries. Talk to your doctor or midwife for more information on safe travel while pregnant.

Talk to Your Doctor about Existing Conditions and Your Family History

If you have any pre-existing conditions, chronic problems or a family history of reproductive problems, you should let your doctor or midwife know about them so that he/she can take appropriate action. Pre-existing conditions include things such as diabetes, herpes (and other sexually transmitted diseases), heart problems, epilepsy and high blood pressure.

Things You Should NOT Do

Smoke or Be Around People Who Do

Smoking is such a well-known hazard to the mother that it only follows that it is also harmful to the baby. Yet hundreds of thousands of pregnant women still smoke. Second-hand smoke from smokers who live or work with pregnant women can also affect the foetus. Exposure to smoke can result in spontaneous abortion, pre-term births, low-weight full-term babies, and foetal and infant deaths.

Drink Alcohol

Alcohol has a variety of negative effects on your developing baby depending on the dose and frequency. Foetal Alcohol Syndrome (FAS) is the worst-case scenario, leading to severe retardation and other abnormalities. FAS is linked to birth defects and is the leading known cause of preventable mental retardation. It is characterized by a number of congenital birth defects, which include pre-natal, and post-natal growth deficiency, facial malformations, central nervous system dysfunction, and varying degrees of major organ system malfunctions.

Take Illegal Drugs

In utero drug exposure is associated with an increased rate of low birth weight, central nervous system damage that may delay or impair neurobehavioural development, mild to severe withdrawal effects, and physical malformations such as cleft palate, heart murmurs, eye defects, and abnormalities of facial features and other organ systems among newborns.

Take Prescription Drugs or Over the Counter (OTC) Drugs, Including Aspirin, Unless Told To By Your Doctor or Midwife

Drugs that are considered 'safe' to take when not pregnant can cause devastating effects to a foetus when you are pregnant. If you are even thinking of becoming pregnant, you should discuss the use of any drugs you currently take with your doctor or midwife beforehand. It is recommended *not to take any OTC drugs*, especially during the first eight weeks of pregnancy when the heart, lung, and brain are being formed.

Note: All drugs, prescription or OTC, have risks and are potentially harmful, pregnant or not.

Eat Hot Dogs

Hot dogs have been implicated in several studies. It has also been found that children under the age of five who eat more than one hot dog a week may have an increased risk of cancer, thought to be due to the concentration of nitrates, nitrites and other preservatives.

Take in Excessive Caffeine

Caffeine (found in coffee, black tea, green tea, cola, chocolate, and energy drinks) taken during pregnancy is thought to increase the probability of a child contracting diabetes as well as increased risk of miscarriage, stillbirth and infant death in the first year of life. Try to limit your intake of caffeine to less than one or two cups of coffee or tea per day (see also page 92).

Have Contact with Reptiles

Be sure to tell your doctor if you have any contact with lizards, iguanas, turtles, or snakes as the salmonella virus is transferred through their faeces and can affect your pregnancy. Also, children under the age of five are also at risk for contracting salmonella if they are in contact with reptiles.

Get a Tick Bite

Tick bites open you to the risk of Lyme disease, which can be deadly to your developing baby.

Eat Fish

Fish concentrate methyl mercury, which is known to affect the developing child's brain. Particularly avoid larger fish such as swordfish, shark, tuna and mackerel as they tend to concentrate more toxins due to their larger size and longer lifespan before harvest.

Note: This warning does not apply to fish oil supplements, which have been shown to increase baby's intelligence as well as decrease the likelihood of developing post-partum depression.

Eat Junk Food

The basic problem with junk food is that it fills you up but does not provide vitamins or protein. As your stomach size decreases during pregnancy, junk food takes up room and prevents you from eating the foods you really need for your and your baby's health. It is also usually loaded with preservatives and unhealthy trans-fats. Additionally, artificial sweeteners such as Aspartame and phenylalanine (NutraSweet™) have been linked with altered foetal brain growth.

Take Vitamin A Supplements

By consuming as little as four times the RDA of vitamin A, you greatly increase the risk of having a baby with birth defects or other problems. Exposure during the first trimester is the worst. Natural sources of vitamin A are okay—it is foods that are artificially supplemented that cause the problem, and most foods are. You need to start reading packages to make sure you are not getting too much vitamin A. Other fat-soluble vitamins such as D, E, and K can also accumulate in the body organs and tissues and high-dosage supplementation should be always by discussed with your doctor or midwife.

Have an X-Ray

The risks posed by x-ray exposure are fairly small, such as low-birth weight, with the greatest risk occurring early in the pregnancy. Informing your doctor or dentist of the fact that you are pregnant is probably the best way to control your risk. If the x-ray can be postponed until after the pregnancy, this will eliminate the risk.

Use Microwaves

The developing foetus is particularly vulnerable to excessive microwave radiation. Microwaving food also tends to destroy delicate vitamins and minerals essential for maintaining an optimal pregnancy and microwaving in plastic should *always* be avoided, as there may be leaching of chemicals (especially hormone disruptors) from the plastics into your food.

Use Teflon

The chemical in Teflon coatings (PFOA, PFOS) has been linked to problems with human development (birth defects) and reproduction (infertility). It does not break down in the environment, bioaccumulates, and has been found to cause various cancers and adverse effects. Teflon can be found in a variety of products from clothes, to stain repellents, to cleaning products, to food packaging, to cosmetics and to Scotchguard. The best thing you can do is avoid Teflon as much as possible. Cast iron cookware is safer and you also get some of the iron you need from cooking with it.

Use an Electric Blanket

Electric blankets give off low-level electromagnetic fields, which may be harmful to a developing baby.

Use a Waterbed

The heaters used in waterbeds give off the same electric fields as those found in electric blankets (see previous) and should therefore be avoided for the same reasons. They are also very bad for your spine.

Drink Tap Water, if Possible

Recent studies have shown that drinking unfiltered tap water during the early months of pregnancy can increase your risk of miscarriage. If this concerns you or you have a history of miscarriage, you may want to drink bottled water or invest in a simple water filtration system such as a Brita® water pitcher or discuss the issue with your doctor or midwife. Do not avoid drinking water, however, as it is essential for maintaining a healthy diet (see *Basic Pregnancy Diet*).

Expose Yourself to Pesticides

Pesticides (including insecticides, herbicides, fungicides and so on) can have a variety of effects on your unborn baby depending on the type of chemical, the length and intensity of exposure and the age of the foetus. In general, it is best to avoid exposure to all pesticides. The problem is that pesticide use is extremely widespread in North America. You can be exposed to pesticides in your home (ant and roach bait traps, no-pest strips, household pest control products and services, flea collars on dogs and cats, etc.), in your yard (lawn care services, do-it-yourself herbicides and insecticides on the lawn or garden), in your neighbourhood (especially in rural areas, but also from suburban neighbours spraying their yards), and from various food sources (non-organic fruit, vegetables, and other foods). The most you can do is attempt to avoid these dangers as best you can.

Inhale Fumes from Paint, Paint Thinner, Household Cleaning Products and so on

There are a large number of toxic products and by-products found in the home and yard. As with pesticides, the best you can hope for is educating yourself and trying to limit your exposure.

Allow Your Body Temperature to Rise

There is a potential danger to the developing foetus if your body temperature rises above 102 degrees Fahrenheit or forty degrees Celsius. You can raise your body temperature to this level by getting a fever, by exercising too strenuously, working outside on hot summer days, and so on.

Use a Sauna, Hot Tub or Take Long Hot Baths

Hot tubs and hot baths have a tendency to raise your body temperature and therefore are to be avoided. See the previous item for details.

Clean Cat Litter Boxes. And You Should Avoid Uncooked Meat.

Both cat litter and undercooked meat present the risk of toxoplasmosis, which can cause birth defects. If you have been around cats since childhood, you are most likely already immune to toxoplasmosis, but it is still a good idea to avoid cleaning the litter box while pregnant.

Contract Herpes or Other STD's

Herpes can be transferred to the baby during delivery, and can lead to severe complications. The easiest way to avoid this possibility is to avoid contracting herpes. *Always* practice safe sex, even when pregnant. If you do have herpes (or any other STD), be sure to tell your doctor or midwife.

[Adapted from: http://www.bygpub.com/natural/pregnancy.htm]

7

Basic Pregnancy Diet

When you are pregnant, you need to eat more quality foods than when you are not pregnant.

Although pre-natal vitamins are in routine use during pregnancy, they do not take the place of a healthy balanced diet. To meet your own and your developing baby's needs, choose the following foods:

1. **Calcium:** three to four servings of calcium-rich foods daily from dairy or non-dairy sources. An example of one serving: 250 millilitres/one cup of milk, fifty grams cheese, 175 grams/three-quarters of a cup of yogurt, 250 millilitres/one cup of pudding, 250 millilitres/one cup cottage cheese or one-quarter cup/125 millilitres raw almonds.
2. **Iron:** up to two servings of iron-rich foods daily.
3. **Protein:** two to three servings of fish (choose smaller fish such as sardines more often as they contain less mercury and heavy metals than shark, swordfish, tuna or mackerel), shellfish, eggs, chicken, turkey, lean beef, veal, pork, or alternative proteins (such as beans, legumes, tofu) daily. An example of one serving of protein: one egg, forty-five grams tuna, fifty grams meat, poultry or fish, half a cup of beans, thirty millilitres/two tablespoons peanut butter, or one hundred grams tofu.
4. **Grains:** five to twelve servings (for example, one serving = one slice of bread, one tortilla, half of a bagel or bun, thirty grams of cereal, three-quarters of a cup cooked cereal, four crackers, or half of a cup pasta or rice) of grain products daily. Choose wholegrain and enriched products most often.
5. **Vegetables and Fruit:** strive to eat five to ten servings of vegetables and fruit *daily* including at least two servings of fresh, green leafy

vegetables, at least two servings of those containing vitamin C (shown to lower the risk of pre-eclampsia and helps with iron absorption), and at least one to two additional servings (especially brightly-coloured red, yellow or orange coloured fruits or vegetables). Try not to drink too much juice as it is high in sugar and you miss out on the healthy fibre.

6. Use butter or healthy oil in small quantities. Avoid hydrogenated oils and trans-fats as they are very unhealthy. Considering supplementing with Omega-3 oil such as fish oil during pregnancy as it is associated with increased intelligence in the baby, decreased risk of premature delivery, and decreased incidence of post-partum depression (additionally, the fish becomes purified of any accumulated heavy metals during processing into fish oil).

7. Drink six to eight glasses of water daily (plus soups and juicy fruits and vegetables).

8. Salt your food to taste.

Folate/Folic Acid

Folate is an important vitamin primarily taken to prevent neural tube defects (e.g. spina bifida) in the foetus. It is also important for new cell production and maintenance as well as DNA replication. Folate (folic acid is the synthetic form) is found in beef liver, fortified cereal, black-eyed peas, brussels sprouts, peanuts, spinach, broccoli, dark leafy lettuce, garbanzo beans/chick peas, and avocado. It is recommended that all women planning to conceive take 400 micrograms (0.4 milligrams) daily and it is best taken with food. B complex vitamins help with absorption of folate, especially vitamin B12 (found in lamb's liver, liver pâté, pork, duck, pheasant, eggs, cod, beef, fortified breakfast cereals, yeast extract, and mushrooms).

Note: Do not use yeast extract or Brewer's Yeast if you have or have had a problem with Candida (e.g. yeast infections or thrush).

Iron

Iron is an important mineral that is needed to carry oxygen in your blood to all parts of your body, especially to the growing foetus. There's an increased need for iron during pregnancy to prevent anaemia (deficiency of haemoglobin and therefore the ability to carry oxygen in the red blood cells) due to the increased volume of blood in circulation. Our bodies tend not to absorb iron very efficiently (hence, why commercial iron supplements often cause constipation) and generally animal sources of iron are more readily bioavailable. Vitamin C helps increase the absorption of iron in the diet. Caffeine and bran decrease the absorption of iron. Good food sources of iron include: red meat, shellfish (clams and oysters), beans, peas, spinach, dark leafy greens, dried fruits (apricots, prunes, raisins, dates, figs), prune juice, nuts (sunflower seeds, brazil nuts, almonds, peanuts, sesame seeds), eggs, whole grains (wheat, oats, barley, millet, corn and brown rice), enriched breads and cereals, farina, blackstrap molasses, Brewer's or nutritional yeast, Ovaltine, wheat germ, seaweed (dulse and kelp), and watermelon. Good herb sources include red raspberry leaves, nettle leaves, dandelion leaves, parsley leaves, yellow dock root, and peppermint leaves. The recommended daily allowance of iron is thirty to sixty milligrams.

Anaemia Prevention Formula

Half an ounce/fifteen grams dried nettle leaves
Half an ounce/fifteen grams dried red raspberry leaves
Half an ounce/fifteen grams dried parsley leaves
Half an ounce/fifteen grams dried dandelion leaves
Quarter ounce/seven and half grams peppermint leaves

Place herbs in a half-gallon/two litre jar.
Pour boiling water over to fill the jar and steep for eight hours.
Strain and drink up to four cups daily for one week of each month.
A little honey may be used to sweeten the infusion to taste.

Calcium

Of course, calcium is also mineral and it is vitally important during pregnancy and throughout life! Inadequate calcium during pregnancy is associated with cramps, backache, intense labour and afterbirth pains, pre-eclampsia, high blood pressure, osteoporosis, and tooth decay. Calcium is needed for bone and teeth formation, blood clotting, and healthy nerve and muscle function. Calcium assimilation is governed by weight-bearing exercise, stress, acidity during digestion, availability of vitamins C (found in papaya, guava, black currants, red and green peppers, broccoli, strawberries, kiwi fruit, citrus fruits, cabbage, and cauliflower), A and especially vitamin D, and availability of magnesium and it's ratio to phosphorus in the body. Also needed for ideal calcium absorption are boron, vitamin B6, copper, folic acid, manganese, silica, strontium and zinc. Food combinations that are thought to interfere with absorption of calcium should be avoided such as spinach, chocolate, rhubarb, and Brewer's Yeast. Too much protein, caffeine, and high sugar and salt intake in the diet are also linked to decreased calcium absorption. Ideally strive to take in 1000 to 2000 milligrams of calcium daily. The best food sources of calcium are fish with bones, dairy products, calcium-fortified orange juice, and nuts. Some of the best food sources include goat's milk and goat cheese (easier assimilation than cow's milk for some), salmon, sardines, mackerel, seaweed (especially kelp), legumes (chick peas, dried green peas, lima beans, kidney beans), sesame seeds, sesame salt (gomasio), tahini, nuts (except peanuts), molasses, and dark leafy greens such as turnip tops, beet greens, broccoli, and kale. Organic bones soaked in organic apple cider vinegar release calcium into the acidic vinegar. A tablespoon of this vinegar in a glass of water supplies needed calcium and relieves morning sickness too. Many fruits are rich in calcium (though not as rich as the above foods)—dried dates, figs raisins, prunes, papaya and elderberries are the best sources. The recommended daily amount of calcium is 800 to 1000 milligrams (one cup of cow's milk contains approximately 300 milligrams of calcium).

Note: Do *not* use bone meal or oyster shell tablets as sources of supplemental calcium. They have been found to be high in lead, mercury, cadmium and other toxic metals. If a supplement is to be used, then choose an organic calcium salt such as calcium gluconate, calcium lactate, calcium citrate, calcium amino acid chelate (there are several of these), calcium orotate, calcium aspartate, or calcium ascorbate with vitamin D, magnesium, and the other trace elements listed above for maximum bioavailability and absorption. In addition, the inorganic forms (calcium sulphate, calcium phosphate and calcium carbonate) are poorly absorbed (only five to ten per cent), and require and bind the most acid, which can lead to the malabsorption of protein.

Table of Herbs That Contain Calcium

Herbs that Contain Calcium	Herbs that Contain Calcium and Vitamin D (increase absorption)	Herbs that Contain Calcium and Magnesium (increase absorption)
Red Raspberry Leaf	Alfalfa	Oat Straw
Nettle	Nettle	Kelp
Alfalfa		Nettle
Oat Straw		Horsetail
Dandelion Leaf		Sage
Comfrey		
Peppermint		
Yellow Dock		
Lamb's Quarter		
Chickweed		
Watercress		
Sage		
Red Clover		
Kelp		
Mustard Greens		
Parsley		
Horsetail		
Coltsfoot		
Plantain		
Borage		
Chicory		
Shepherd's Purse		

One large mugful of herbal infusion will give you 250 to 300 milligrams of useable calcium. Adding a small pinch of horsetail to infusion adds ten per cent more calcium (mostly due to the magnesium and silica).

8

Herbs

The best approach with herbs is the regular use of tonics to prevent problems.

For example, prepared as a tea or an infusion, the nutrients provided in the plant are better assimilated than in the harder-to-digest capsule form. Teas can be used to increase the supply of vitamins and minerals, increase energy, and improve uterine tone. Teas and infusions can be taken hot, chilled or at room temperature.

To prepare tea: infuse one to three teaspoons/five to fifteen grams of the dried or fresh herb in a cup of boiling water and steep for ten to fifteen minutes. A bodum or coffee plunger pot works well, or one can strain out the loose herbs later (a tea ball frequently doesn't allow the water to permeate and surround the herbs very well).

To make infusion of leaves: pour one quart/one litre of boiling water over one-ounce/thirty grams for a minimum of four hours. Cap the jar and then strain in the morning. Drink some every day. This is especially effective for calcium-containing herbs.

To make infusion of flowers: one-ounce/thirty grams in one quart/one litre of water for two hours minimum.

To prepare mineral vinegar: infuse vinegar (use organic apple cider vinegar) with some of the herbs for a month and take at least one-tablespoon/fifteen millilitres a day and/or use it in cooking. The acidity helps your body absorb the minerals through your stomach.

Herbs Used Safely In Pregnancy

Red Raspberry Leaf (Rubus idaeus)

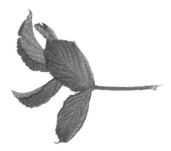

Typically brewed as a tea or as an infusion (red raspberry tea ice cubes are great to suck on during labour), red raspberry leaves are the best known, most widely used, and safest of all uterine/pregnancy tonic herbs. Rubus can be used throughout pregnancy, but is particularly useful in the third trimester. Most of the benefits ascribed to regular use of this plant throughout pregnancy can be traced to the presence of the strengthening power of the alkaloid, fragrine, and/or to the nourishing power of the vitamins and minerals. Rich in vitamin C, vitamin E, easily assimilated calcium and iron, as well as vitamin A and B complex and many other minerals including phosphorus and potassium. Benefits of drinking red raspberry leaf brew include: easing morning sickness, helping prevent miscarriage and post-partum haemorrhage due to poor uterine tone, tonifying the muscles of the pelvic region including the uterus itself, coordinating uterine contractions for a speedier, easier birth, reducing labour and after-birth pains, and it can help increase breast milk production.

Note: Red raspberry leaf is also an excellent herb for increasing fertility, especially when combined with red clover (see also *Appendix Three—A Plausible Cause of Infertility Discovered*).

Nettle Leaf (Urtica dioica)

The taste of this infusion is deep and rich and nettle leaves are known as one of the finest nourishing tonics. It has more chlorophyll than any other herb (even more than algae) and nearly every vitamin and mineral necessary for human health and growth. Especially abundant in nettle are vitamins A, C, D and K, calcium, potassium, phosphorus, iron and sulphur. Benefits of drinking nettle infusion before and during pregnancy include: aiding the kidneys with elimination, detoxification, nourishing mother and foetus, easing leg cramps and other muscle spasms due to the calcium, diminishing pain during and after birth, preventing haemorrhage after birth due to the vitamin K, reducing haemorrhoids, tightening and strengthening blood vessels thereby reducing broken capillaries and varicose veins, and increasing the amount and richness of breast milk.

Note: Some pregnant women alternate weeks of nettle and red raspberry brews; others drink raspberry until the last month and then switch to nettles to insure large amounts of vitamin K in the blood before birth.

Dandelion Leaf (Taraxacum officinale)

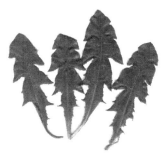

Dandelion leaf is a good source of calcium and potassium in addition to vitamins A, B1, B2, C and D, iron, zinc, choline and many trace minerals. This tea vitalizes and heals the liver, promotes bile production in the gall bladder, and also helps the kidneys function better. Dandelion leaves are vitally important in the prevention and treatment of pregnancy-related oedema, pre-eclampsia, and it can help restore a slow moving digestive tract. Fresh (best picked when the dandelion rosette first emerges, before flowering) or dried dandelion herbs are also used as a mild appetite stimulant and to improve upset stomach (such as feelings of fullness, flatulence, and constipation). The root of the dandelion plant is believed to have mild laxative effects and is often used to improve digestion. Chinese medicine practitioners traditionally used dandelion to treat digestive disorders, appendicitis, and breast problems (such as inflammation or lack of milk flow). Dandelion leaves can also be used to help with premenstrual symptoms, particularly water retention.

Note: Dandelion root is often also used as a bitter to raise low spirits.

Alfalfa (Medicago sativa)

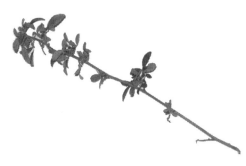

Alfalfa helps increase the availability of vitamin K and haemoglobin in the blood thereby preventing haemorrhage as well as encouraging a good breast milk supply. It can also aid in elimination from a slow moving digestive tract. Alfalfa is a good laxative and a natural diuretic; it alkalizes and detoxifies the body, especially the liver. It also promotes pituitary gland function and contains an anti-fungus agent. The Chinese have used alfalfa since the sixth century to treat kidney stones, and to relieve fluid retention and swelling. Alfalfa contains vitamins A, B1, B2, D, E, and K. The leaves of the alfalfa plant are rich in minerals and nutrients, including calcium, magnesium, potassium, chlorophyll, and carotene (useful against both heart disease and cancer).

Oat Straw (Avena sativa)

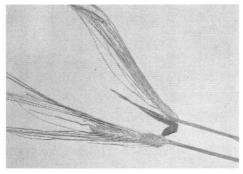

Oat straw is used to strengthen the capillaries and prevent varicosities and haemorrhoids. It is good for the heart, nerves, insomnia, indigestion, and is often used in homeopathic remedies. Benefits of consistent use of oats and oat straw in the diet: reduces cholesterol and improves circulatory function, helps to stabilize blood sugar levels, brings about noticeable improvement in coordination, bone density, balance, memory, sensitivity to pleasant stimuli, clarity of thinking, overall calmness, and centeredness. Oat straw is also one of the best remedies for "feeding" the nervous system. Oat straw is a nervine, that strengthens nerves, helps people deal with stress due to the vitamin B complex, maintains restful sleep patterns, reduces the frequency and duration of headaches, and is useful for menopausal symptoms (particularly insomnia, depression, anxiety, memory loss, restless legs). The high level of silicic acid in the straw explains its use as a remedy for skin conditions, especially externally. The nutritive properties of oats and oat straw are not very different, except that oat straw is lower in calories and higher in vitamin A (carotene) and vitamin C, than the grain alone. Oat straw is also high in calcium, phosphorus, vitamins B1, B2, A and E.

Slippery Elm (Ulmus fulva)

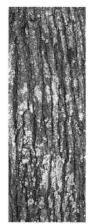

Native Americans traditionally used slippery elm as a poultice for boils, ulcers, and for wounds in general. Internally, it was commonly used for colds or fevers, and to soothe an irritated digestive system—one of its main uses today. The 'slippery' part of slippery elm refers to the texture of the herb. This is because of the large mucilage content of slippery elm, which is also responsible for its wonderful healing and soothing action. It not only soothes and heals all that it comes into contact with, but is highly nutritious. Slippery elm is a wholesome food for the weak and convalescent, from infants to the elderly. Taken internally, slippery elm can be used to help soothe many different types of digestive complaints. For example: irritable bowel syndrome (IBS), colitis and diverticulitis, inflammation of the gut or colic, can give instant relief to heartburn or 'reflux', (this is a common use for slippery elm in pregnancy), ulcers anywhere in the gut (stomach and intestines), and diarrhoea (especially if mixed with a banana and powdered marshmallow root). It can also be useful for urinary infections such as cystitis. Traditionally, slippery elm is also reported to ease chest, lung, and bronchial conditions. To make powder/tea drink: mix one teaspoon of herb with a little water to a paste. Slowly add half a pint/250 millilitres or so of boiling water, stirring or whisking all the time. Drink two to three cups daily or follow the instructions on the package.

Cramp Bark (Viburnum opulus)

Cramp bark is particularly useful if there is spotting in the early stages of pregnancy and to prevent miscarriage due to stress and anxiety (use only under the supervision of a health care provider). Although cramp bark contains small amounts of several different types of compounds, a chemical known as viopudial is believed to provide cramp bark with its cramp-relieving effects. Viopudial is thought to relax muscles by partially blocking an enzyme involved with causing muscle spasms. It may also have direct effects on muscle tissue—particularly the muscles in the uterus. Although one of the traditional uses of cramp bark has been to relax the uterus when uterine muscle spasms threaten to cause a miscarriage, it may complicate pregnancy. Cramp bark is also used for painful menstrual cramps. Decoction: put two teaspoonfuls of the dried bark into a cup of water and bring to the boil. Simmer gently for ten to fifteen minutes. This should be drunk hot three times a day. Tincture: take four to eight millilitres of the tincture, three times a day.

Black Haw (Viburnum prunifolium)

Black haw may be used under the supervision of a health care provider in the early stages of pregnancy to help prevent miscarriage. It has similar uses to its relative, cramp bark. It is a powerful uterine relaxant and is used in the treatment of spasmodic dysmenorrhoea (painful menstruation), excessive menstrual flow (especially around menopause), and false labour pains. It may be used for threatened miscarriage as well. It is used to treat vaginal and cervical discharges. Its relaxant and sedative actions explain its ability to reduce blood pressure, which is achieved through relaxation of the peripheral blood vessels. It may be used as an antispasmodic in the treatment of asthma. A cream may be applied to muscle cramps or muscle tension. It acts as a uterine tonic, sedative, nervine, spasmolytic, anti-asthmatic, hypotensive, anti-diarrhoeal, and astringent.

Pregnancy Brew

Half an ounce/fifteen grams dried red raspberry leaves
Half an ounce/fifteen grams dried nettle leaves
Quarter ounce/seven and half grams dried dandelion leaves
Quarter ounce/ seven and half grams dried alfalfa
Quarter ounce/ seven and half grams dried oat straw

Place herbs in a half-gallon/two litre jar.
Pour boiling water over to fill the jar and steep for eight hours.
Strain and drink up to two cups daily.
A little honey may be used to sweeten the brew to taste.

9

Herbs To Use With CAUTION during Pregnancy and Breastfeeding

1. **Squaw Vine (Mitchella repens), Blue Cohosh (Caulophyllum thalicotroides)**, and **Black Cohosh (Cimicifuga racemosa)** should all be avoided until the last four to six weeks of pregnancy as they are uterine stimulants. Even then, they should be used only when indicated, and under the supervision of someone experienced in their use. Some midwives report that the Cohoshes must be used together (not interchangeably). Others have reported premature labour when Blue Cohosh was taken in combination with Pennyroyal.
2. Some people feel that **Comfrey (Symphytum officinale)** is not safe to use during pregnancy. The roots of Comfrey do contain compounds that are best avoided during pregnancy (as do all parts of the wild plant). In fact, Comfrey root may cause liver congestion in mother and baby. One of the uses of Comfrey Leaf that is considered safe is in a sitz bath post-partum (see section titled *"Returning the Uterus, Perineum and Abdominal Muscles to Normal More Quickly"* for more information).
3. **Chamomile** may cause allergic reactions in susceptible women. Avoid if you develop symptoms of allergy or know you have an allergy to Chamomile.

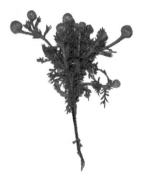

4. Another important herbal ally for women over forty who desire a child is **Chaste Tree (Vitex agnus-casti)**. It has been used in Africa and parts of Europe for several thousand years to discourage the male libido. In women, the effects seem to be the opposite! It may also be a fertility enhancer. Most importantly, chaste tree is a strengthening tonic for the pituitary gland, the master control gland for the endocrine system. Daily use of the tincture of the berries (one dropperful/one millilitres two to three times daily) had been shown to increase progesterone (the hormone of pregnancy) and luteinizing hormone (which promotes conception). Because it can lower prolactin levels, chaste tree is best discontinued during the last trimester of pregnancy.

5. **Ginseng (Panax ginseng)** should not be taken during pregnancy unless administered by a practitioner of Chinese Medicine and monitored closely. Side effects may include lowering blood sugar levels.

6. **Licorice root, St. John's wort, Motherwort,** and **Vitex** should only be used with caution and under medical supervision during pregnancy and breastfeeding.

10

Herbs to AVOID during Pregnancy and Breastfeeding

1. **Dong quai (Angelica sinensis)** is not recommended for women over forty. In general, this herb promotes blood flow to the uterus and surrounding tissues. This can promote the growth of fibroids and increase the risk of post-partum haemorrhage. It can also stimulate suppressed menstruation. Ginger is a better warming tonic; motherwort is better at relieving pain; and red raspberry leaf is better at preparing the uterus for birth.
2. **CoEnzyme Q10 supplements** are best avoided during pregnancy unless an urgent medical problem warrants its use (e.g. a heart condition and then only under the supervision of a doctor) as the potential side effects are not known.
3. **False Unicorn Root (Helonias dioica), Pennyroyal,** and **PN6 capsules** are considered too strong for use during pregnancy.
4. **Goldenseal (Hydrastis canadenis)** should *not* be taken during pregnancy, as it is an alkaloid-containing herb, which may cause harm to the baby or cause miscarriage.
5. **Borage Oil** and **Fenugreek** should not be used during pregnancy, as they are uterine stimulants. They are useful during lactation to increase milk supply (see *Breastfeeding Problems* section).
6. **Blessed Thistle** should also be avoided during pregnancy as it may cause vomiting in high doses (see also *Breastfeeding Problems* section).
7. **Henbane, Elder, Mugwort, Nutmeg** (may cause miscarriage in high doses), **Rue, Saffron, Yarrow, Devil's Claw, Scothbroom, Marigold, Ragweed, Juniper Berries, Buckthorn Bark, Senna Leaves, Duck Roots, Aloe** (taken internally), **Sassafras Root, Tansy, Cotton Root Bark, Angelica** (may stimulate bleeding), **Cascara Sagrada, Calamus Root, Foxglove, Lily of the Valley, Oleander, Squill, Ma Huang** (also known as **ephedra, ephedrine, Mormon Tea** or **Desert Tea**) and **Uva Ursi** should all be avoided during pregnancy.

11

Homeopathy

Homeopathy is a natural system of health care developed by German chemist Samuel Hahnemann (1755-1843).

Homeopathy utilises plant, mineral, animal and metals to trigger the body's vital force to heal itself. Homeopathy stresses the importance of looking at the whole state of the person to find the most beneficial remedy in a given circumstance. Homeopathic remedies (also called homeopathics) are a system of medicine based on three principles:

- **Like Cures Like (the Law of Similars)**

For example, if the symptoms of your cold were similar to poisoning by mercury, then mercury would be your homeopathic remedy.

- **Minimal Dose**

The remedy is taken in an extremely dilute form, using serial dilutions. For example, a 1X dose is one part per nine parts liquid, a 30C dose is one part per 99 parts liquid, and a 1M dose is one part per 999 parts liquid. Generally, the more dilute the remedy, the more potent it is. Particularly in pregnancy and labour it is best to use a higher potency remedy (e.g. a 200C versus a 30C). You may need to speak to your midwife, a homeopath or another health care provider to obtain a 200C or 1M dose as they are not always readily available in health food stores.

- **The Single Remedy**

No matter how many symptoms are experienced, only one remedy is taken, and that remedy will be aimed at all those symptoms.

Similar principals form the basis of conventional allergy treatment, where the allergic substance is given in a small dose, and in vaccines where an impotent form of the virus is given to bolster the immune system against that particular virus.

Homeopathic remedies can be extremely effective and are safe to use in pregnant women and babies but the catch is that exactly the right remedy needs to be taken for your symptoms. With the sheer number of remedies available, this can be a daunting and difficult task! The most common remedies will be covered here and if you find that a particular remedy is not working for you, you have probably not chosen the right one for the condition in conjunction with your constitution, and should consult a classical homeopath for advice. Also, it is best to dissolve the remedy under your tongue, and to not eat or drink anything twenty minutes before and twenty minutes after taking it for maximum effectiveness.

Homeopathic Remedies Safely Used in Pregnancy:

Nausea, Vomiting

Sepia

The personality/mood characteristics associated with Sepia are:

- worse from the smell or thought of food, better if eats a little food;
- generally are quite ambivalent to loved ones, irritable;
- want to be left alone, quiet, don't want another responsibility, may have guilt;
- marked poor memory and poor concentration;
- heavy feeling in perineum (feels as if the uterus will fall out) even in the beginning of pregnancy;
- can have extreme anger, low libido, doesn't want to be touched;
- vigorous motion may make her feel better in the early stages; and
- constipation and cold sensitivity may be present.

Ipecac

The personality/mood characteristics associated with Ipecac are:

- terrible nausea, unrelieved by vomiting, quite extreme;
- quite irritable, profuse salivation, thirstless;
- pink tongue (not coated);
- worse in a warm room or with motion;
- better in the open air (e.g. ideal is sitting or resting with an open window); and
- nose bleeds (bleeds easily).

Pulsatilla

The personality/mood characteristics associated with Pulsatilla are:

- sensitive, yielding disposition, weepy;
- wants company (not to be left alone), consolation;
- stools vary from loose to hard or constipated;
- variability in temperament (sweet irritability);
- want fresh air, love slow walks in the fresh air;
- sensitive to rich and fatty foods but may crave butter, cream; and
- very thirstless.

Note: You can also use Pulsatilla for breech or transverse lies *after thirty-six weeks* if other adjustments (e.g. chiropractic, Hypnobirthing®) didn't work. You need to use a 200C or 1M dose three times a day for three to four doses, then two times per day for a couple of days. Pulsatilla can also be used for heartburn if the food feels stuck behind your breastbone, your tongue is coated and you crave starchy foods, which make the symptoms worse. Dose is 30C every two hours.

Phosphorus

The personality/mood characteristics associated with Phosphorus are:

- bubbly, extroverted person;
- possibly fearful, worried;
- sympathetic, caring, very likeable;

- loves ice cold drinks, very thirsty, and may like carbonated drinks;
- vomits twenty minutes after having a cold drink (once liquid has warmed up in the stomach);
- can feel chilly (cold); and
- can have burning sensations (e.g. heartburn).

Tabacum

The personality/mood characteristics associated with Tabacum are:

- dizzy, vertigo, lots of saliva (spitting);
- better from vomiting, better from cool air;
- better from keeping eyes closed (worse with eyes open); and
- worse with motion.

Colchicum

The personality/mood characteristics associated with Colchicum are:

- more sensitive to smells than Sepia (foods, perfumes, car exhaust etc.);
- a lot of saliva and spitting it out;
- worse with motion; and
- chilly (better with warmth and rest).

Vaginitis

(pH balance in the vagina is skewed)

Pulsatilla

- go with the Pulsatilla mental/emotional state under *Nausea, Vomiting* section as well as symptoms including: copious bland discharge (thick, yellow, creamy), itchy and foul but not burning, and possibly irritating.

Sepia

- go with the Sepia mental/emotional state under *Nausea, Vomiting* section as well as the following symptoms: the vulva will feel raw and irritated, possibly have lesions, there is a feeling of heaviness in perineum, and mother feels better with exercise.

Caulophyllum

- profuse irritating discharge, more towards the end of pregnancy, chilly, irritated, nervous (high strung), and weak. May bring on labour or prevent miscarriage depending on when used (consult your homeopathic practitioner).

Kreosotum

- use in severe cases of vaginitis: foul, burning, stings when urinating, lots of itching and swelling, irritable disposition, and mother wants cold on the perineum and vulva.

Varicosities

Pulsatilla

- go with Pulsatilla mental/emotional state under *Nausea, Vomiting* section.

Sepia

- go with Sepia mental/emotional state under *Nausea, Vomiting* section.

Hamamelis (Witch Hazel)

- delicate veins, congestion, sore and stingy sensation, and is a great remedy for haemorrhoids too.

Lachesis

- use when varicosities are worse on the left side, mother is sensitive to touch and constriction (wants nothing tight on legs, waist and especially the neck), legs can be purple, worse in hot weather, better with cool air, quite chatty/talkative, better with discharge (e.g. talking, crying), better from food, worse from saliva, and worse during sleep or after sleep.

Note: Lachesis is also good for sore throats, especially ones that are worse on the left.

Labour Helpers

Caulophyllum (Blue Cohosh)

- use for threatened miscarriage and delayed maturity (post-due date). Mother may be nervous, excitable, easily displeased. Labour doesn't really kick in: feeble, irregular contractions, uterus feels congested, sluggish, with no sustained effort, with no regular rhythm, and labour pains are short, irregular and spasmodic (short, crampy, intermittent, more in groin and bladder). Patient may feel exhausted, and can scarcely speak at times. There tends to be a rigid cervical os (opening) with very little dilation, and possibly needle-like sensations around the cervix. Dose: 200C every couple of hours for three to four doses then wait twenty-four hours (then go for a brisk walk and make love!).

Cimicifuga (Black Cohosh)

- mother has a sense of gloominess, morose, possibly some hysteria, possibly a bad past birth experience, agitated, feels something bad is going to happen (e.g. feels she is going insane), fragmentation, and possible chattiness. Mother may feel chilly, sensitive to noise and is better with warmth. Contractions go from side to side, more violent, and are predominantly in the lower uterine segment. The cervix is rigid and closed with changeable dilation.

Gelsemium (Yellow Jasmine)

- use if mother is excited in anticipation of the "first" baby and baby is post-due date. Mother may have performance anxiety, chattering teeth, nervousness, thirstlessness, and possible muscle weakness and achiness. Dose: 200C.

Pulsatilla

- use in cases of post-maturity where mother has a mild, weepy, sweet, 'don't leave me,' needing lots of reassurance mental state (e.g. under *Nausea/Vomiting* section).

Aconite

- use if mother had a frightening experience with a past birth (e.g. feel as if they are going to die) and is afraid, restless, and panicky. The mother may be anxious, short of breath, have heart palpitations, have a flushed face (showing emotion in the face), and be thirsty for cold drinks. This remedy is particularly used in the transition stage of labour or if labour progresses to a certain place and then gets stuck due to fear. Use this remedy when energy is stagnant, things aren't happening and/or if the baby isn't quite happy (e.g. showing irregular respiration).

Kalicarbonicum (Potash)

-   use when baby has a posterior presentation: sharp, cutting, severe pains and pressure on the mother's back. Pain is in the sacrum to the buttocks and the thighs. Generally the mother is better from walking and pressure on the sacrum. This remedy is best used in the late first stage and early second stage of labour. Dose: 200C every ten minutes.

Chamomilla (Chamomile)

-   sometimes called the "morphine of pregnancy" and can be used if mother is angry, demanding and ordering people around, and intolerant of pain. Quite often the mother will demand to be taken to the hospital with planned home births. Mother can be nasty, bitchy, abusive, short-tempered, doesn't want to be touched, and is having a hard time with the pain. Mother is better with fresh air and movement, can be thirstless so remember to encourage drinking.

Note: Chamomilla is good for calming teething infants or capricious, cranky toddlers (e.g. ask for things then don't want it)!

Nux Vomica (Poison Nut)

-   use if the bladder is full and mother can't go or bladder/rectum is/feels obstructed. Mother may have the urge to urinate but can't go or can have spasming of the urinary sphincter and you don't want to catheterize. Mother may be irritable, impatient, sensitive to light, noise and odours. The labour pains are felt extending to the back and rectum.

Note: Nux Vomica is also used as a hangover remedy. And for heartburn associated with heaviness after meals, excess gas and a bitter taste in the mouth. Dose is 30C every couple of hours until you feel better.

Belladonna

- use when there is a sudden, violent onset to labour when the contractions come and go suddenly, especially on the right side. The cervix is swollen, rigid and there is no dilation in the first stage. Mother may be headachy, sensitive to jarring, have a red face, she may be hot, have dilated pupils, and may have a wild-eyed expression on her face.

Note: Belladonna is also good for children with fevers.

Coffea Cruda (Unroasted Coffee)

- use when the mother faints due to pain and hyper-excitement of the nervous system, mother has an oversensitivity to pain, all of mother's senses are more acute, the pain is experienced in the small of her back, and mother may cry out or scream with extreme fear.

General Note: Multiple remedies can be used in labour if needed.

Haemorrhoids

Hamamelis (Witch Hazel)

- use if the symptoms of the haemorrhoids include bleeding, bruising, soreness, aching, and tenderness.

Pulsatilla

- use if the appropriate mental/emotional state under *Nausea/Vomiting* section accompanies the haemorrhoids.

Sepia

- use if the appropriate mental/emotional state under *Nausea/Vomiting* section applies as well as a heavy, sagging feeling or a sensation of a 'ball in the rectum' accompanies the haemorrhoids.

Nux Vomica

- use if eating/craving rich food, constipation, and irritability accompany the haemorrhoids.

Sulphur

- use if symptoms include itching, a hot, burning pain that is worse after a bath, if the mother is better using cold compresses and is thirsty for cold drinks.

Lachesis

- use if the haemorrhoids are worse with tight clothing, worse on the left side, worse after sleeping and/or have a blue-purple discolouration.

Aesculus (Horse Chestnut)

- use this remedy if there is a sensation of 'sticks' or prickles in the rectum, no bleeding, and a burning pain, possibly radiating to the hips and back.

Collinsonia (Stone Root)

- use if the symptoms are similar to the Sepia mental/emotional state with constipation, a 'sticks' sensation in the rectum, and possibly bleeding.

Homeopathic Remedies Safely Used Post-Partum

Arnica Montana (Mountain Daisy)

- use to promote healing from trauma (soft tissue injuries, swelling, lacerations, contusions (bruising), tears), encourages the resorption of blood, and prevents infection. It also encourages good uterine tone after birth and can help with remedying overexertion from labour (e.g. when the whole chest wall feels bruised). Arnica can be used for a sore abdomen from an overactive baby or in the case of threatened miscarriage especially after car accidents or falls. Arnica is also useful to speed healing in the baby in the case of caput (swollen head), misshapen head, bruising, and bloodshot eyes, especially if there has been a long second stage of labour. Dose for infants: crush a couple of pellets and use in liquid dilution every fifteen minutes for three doses.

Note: Do NOT take Arnica *before* surgery or dental treatments as it can increase the tendency to haemorrhage.

Hypericum (St. John's Wort)

-   use for lacerations, tears, sharp pains (possible nerve damage), pain shooting in different directions, and can be used in conjunction with Arnica. This remedy is particularly effective with tailbone injuries and whiplash.

Staphysagria

-   use when there are surgical cuts and a lot of pain.

Aconite

-   use for the baby when there has been a rough second stage of labour and there is shallow, rapid respiration (baby isn't really here yet/not settling in). A 30C dose is useful in this case. Aconite is also used if there is retained urine post-partum.

Causticum

-   use if there is retained urine in mother or baby with a numb sensation. The urine may dribble instead of a full stream. A 30C dose is used.

General Note: A wonderful soothing and healing remedy that is sprayed on the vulva when going to the washroom can be made from Arnica, Hypericum and Calendula tincture mixed with filtered water.

Conjunctivitis

Use breast milk in the baby's eye when you are taking these remedies:

Pulsatilla

-   use when there is no redness, just thick, goopy, bland discharge in the baby's eye that may be yellow-green in colour.

Sulphur

-   use when there is thick, yellow-green coloured discharge with eye redness (blood shot appearance and red conjunctiva) and burning.

Mucus in the Baby's Lungs

Crush a couple pellets and mix with filtered water. Give a couple drops of liquid dilution to baby every couple hours.

Aconite

-   use first.

Antimonium Tart

-   use if baby hasn't expelled the mucus and breathing is sounding 'rattley' after day two to three.

Homeopathic Remedies Used for Breastfeeding Problems

Pulsatilla

-   helpful with hormonal regulation in conjunction with the appropriate mental state and can dry up milk or restore it if blocked by mastitis. Dose: use three doses in twenty-four hours: 30C, 12C and then 9C.

Lac Caninum (Dog's Milk)

-   can be used to augment or restore milk production and to reduce the pain of engorgement.

Lac Defloratum (Cow's Milk)

-   can be used to increase or decrease milk production (does what you need) and can increase the quality of milk with proper sucking from the baby.

Calendula Ointment

-   use for cracked, sore nipples, also for soreness with nursing.

Castor Equi

-   use for deep cracks, ulcerations and soreness in the nipples.

Hepar Sulph

- use for deep cracks, sore, painful nipples that are pus-filled or infected. May smell like old cheese (purulent odour).

Note: Hepar Sulph is a good remedy for boils and abscesses.

Silica

- use when there are sharp, splinter-like pains when the baby nurses.

Mastitis

Belladonna

- especially useful if there is rapid onset with redness (or red streaks), the inflammation is on the right breast, mother is restless and sensitive to touch and jarring. There may be throbbing pains and heat in the breast.

Bryonia (Wild Hops)

- use when there is a slower onset breast infection that is worse from motion (e.g. want to wear a bra and want to support the breast). Often the mother will lie on the same side as the infection and the breast is stony-hard. The mother generally wants to be left alone, is irritable, is thirsty for cold drinks, and is better with fresh air. Wait twenty-four hours before changing remedies if this remedy is used.

Phytolacca (Poke Root Berries)

- use Belladonna and Bryonia first as this is a glandular remedy, used when the whole body is involved and the pain in the breast(s) radiates out. The breast(s) is heavy and stony hard. The milk can coagulate, become stringy, and can hang from the nipples. Glands (lymph nodes) in the armpit and neck can also be raised. Dose: every two hours for four to five doses then wait twenty-four hours before changing the remedy.

Silica

- mother may feel chilly, weak, and sensitive to drafts and cold air with the breast abscess. The nipples are cracked and the old lumps possibly haven't completely healed. Dose: three to four doses and give it thirty-six hours to work.

Note: Silica also works for children that are sick and/or get abscesses a lot.

Hepar Sulph

- use when the mother feels chilly, cold, irritable, and there is infection/pus-formation. The mother will want warm drinks and warm compresses.

12

Natural Remedies for Specific Pregnancy, Post-Partum and Newborn Conditions

Softening of Bones and Joints

(e.g. Low Back Pain, Sore Hips and Knees)

- Chiropractic, massage, deep heating rub (e.g. Tiger Balm), and/or acupuncture can help.
- Get regular gentle exercise and stretching (see *An Expectant Parent's Guide to Chiropractic—Pregnancy Exercise Tips* section).
- Drink lemon juice in water up to six glasses a day to cleanse the kidneys.
- Take calcium (see *Table of Herbs Containing Calcium*).
- Avoid excess meat and sugar as this interferes with calcium absorption.
- Use nettle leaf tea.
- If there are muscle spasms, also try St. John's wort or skullcap.
- Use a body pillow for sleeping that you can bunch for support as needed.

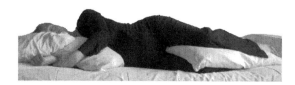

- Use an abdominal support band (also called a "belly bra").
- Hydrotherapy can also bring relief. Use sixty seconds of hot water and then thirty seconds cold shower on the lower pelvis (below the belly) and lower back. Alternate three times and finish with cold water. Repeat this treatment twice a day (in the morning and in the evening).

Note: Pregnant women should avoid excessive heat or steam, so do not use a hot tub or sauna as the high temperatures may harm the baby.

- Use good posture and body mechanics (see *How to Care For Your Spine—Good Pregnancy Body Mechanics* section).
- Keep your weight evenly distributed on both feet when standing.
- If you have to stand for extended periods of time, you may try to shift your weight from one foot to the other for brief periods. Using a small box or step stool (or open your cupboard under the sink and use the lowest shelf) to alternate putting one foot up then the other may also help. Also try to walk around.
- Always squat down and use your legs to lift. You should never lift with your back, even when you're not pregnant! Keep your back straight. Do NOT bend from the waist.
- Encourage young children and toddlers to climb on a stool or chair so that you don't have to pick them up from the floor.
- Do pelvic rocking:

  ◊ Standing—lift the abdomen up while tucking your buttocks under.
  ◊ Lying on your back—bend your knees, place your feet on the floor (or bed) and flatten your lower back against the floor (or bed). Your buttocks should rise a little. Hold this for a few seconds, remembering to breathe, and then relax. Repeat several times.
  ◊ On your hands and knees—inhale and stretch your head up, relax your back (but do NOT let it sway in). Exhale and stretch/arch the back up (like an angry cat).

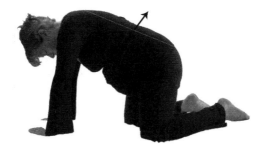

Note: This pose is VERY helpful for back labour. It can also be done leaning on a birthing ball with your arms/chest for support.

- See *Chiropractic* section and *Chart of Effects of Spinal Misalignments* for more information.

Round Ligament Pain

- Moving too quickly (e.g. getting out of bed or sneezing) may stretch ligaments that support your uterus and cause a sharp pain in the lower abdomen.
- To avoid this pain, move slowly, especially getting out of bed. Slowly roll over to your side. Push up with your arms and swing your feet over the edge of the bed so that your abdominal and lower back muscles are not strained.

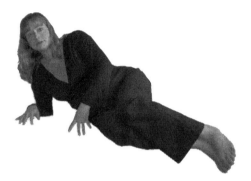

- If you experience round ligament pain, lean toward the affected side, take a deep breath, then relax as much as possible.

Headaches

- Very common in the first trimester of pregnancy due to hormonal changes.
- Try chiropractic, massage, deep heating rub applied to the muscles of the neck and/or acupuncture (See *Chiropractic* section and *Chart of Effects of Spinal Misalignments* for more information).
- Use an ergonomic pillow that supports the curve of the neck.
- Avoid taking anti-inflammatories such as aspirin or ibuprofen as these have been found to increase the risk of miscarriage by up to eighty per cent (even when taken up to three months prior to becoming pregnant).

Note: If the headaches persist after the twenty-eighth week of pregnancy, and are accompanied by water retention, and/or an increase in blood pressure contact your health care provider immediately.

Nasal Stuffiness

- Sniffing warm salt water or using saline nasal spray can help.
- Use a vaporizer at night/humidifier during the day.
- Use Breathe Right Strips on your nose at night.
- Try mentholated natural cough drops (preferably ones without artificial sweeteners).
- Try herbal nasal inhalants (sold at health and natural foods stores).
- Avoid eating excess dairy and other foods that you are sensitive to (food sensitivity testing is available at most Naturopathic Doctor's offices or by seeing an allergy specialist).

Preventing Stretch Marks

- Add twenty drops of mandarin orange and five drops of jasmine essential oils to four ounces/125 millilitres of cocoa butter, unscented lotion or massage oil. Massage your belly, breasts (and other areas that are stretching) daily after a shower or bath while the skin is still damp. This is best used from the fourth month onwards.
- Don't eat for two (adults), which may cause you to gain weight too quickly! It is best to eat very well for one and add only about 300 *quality* extra calories per day (mainly to come from good sources of protein). An average weight gain of 12.7 kilograms (twenty-eight pounds) (or a range of ten to fifteen kilograms (twenty-two to thirty-five pounds)) is considered ideal (see the section titled *Basic Pregnancy Diet* for more information). Maternal obesity is associated with an increased risk of pre-eclampsia, diabetes, increased risk of having to deliver by caesarean section, delivering an abnormally large baby, increased risk of certain structural birth defects, and carrying the baby longer than usual (see the *References* and *Resources* section for all the studies on the risks associated with maternal obesity).

Varicosities and Haemorrhoids

- Avoid commercial preparations such as Preparation H or Anusol as they contain local anaesthetics and mercury and should not be used during pregnancy as they may harm the baby
- Eat beets, oats (e.g. granola), buckwheat, leafy green vegetables (e.g. spinach), okra, wheat germ, dandelion, raw garlic, onions, lecithin, oat straw, nettle leaves, and parsley leaves
- See *Homeopathy* section.

- Increase your fibre intake, and avoid straining during bowel movements.
- Swimming and brisk walking are excellent exercises for increasing your circulation and aiding digestion.
- Support stockings can be helpful if you have to do a lot of standing and you have a tendency towards varicose veins. Elevate your legs for five to ten minutes before putting them on.
- Avoid tight clothing, knee-high stockings, crossing your legs and sitting in one position for too long at a time (e.g. sitting in the car).
- A five-minute leg massage daily can be helpful (and feels great!). Work upwards towards the heart with the flow of the veins and try not to work too hard in order to avoid causing bruising.
- Leg inversions can also help prevent and provide some relief from varicose veins. Lie on your back on the floor close to a wall (your buttocks should touch the wall) and legs going up the wall. Wiggle your toes and rotate your ankles periodically. This can be done for ten to fifteen minutes a day as long as you are comfortable (sometimes lying on your back can cause an increase or decrease in blood pressure during pregnancy so discontinue if you feel dizzy or otherwise uncomfortable). Another position that works is lying on your back on the floor and propping your legs up on the couch, a chair or the bed with a gentle bend in the knees (avoid having the chair etc. press into the back of the knees as this may impede blood flow)
- Use alcohol-free baby wipes to gently keep the vulva/anal area very clean.
- Increase your intake of vitamin E (wheat germ oil, sunflower seeds, almonds, hazelnuts, pine nuts, avocado, sweet potato, and/or take the d-alpha tocopherol form of the vitamin E supplement as the dl-alpha tocopherol is not as effective). Up to 600 IU daily is considered safe during pregnancy.

Note: Vitamin E supplements should be ceased at least two weeks prior to the due date as it may cause the placenta to adhere to the uterine wall more tightly (e.g. makes it "sticky").

- Apply witch hazel cream externally, or use distilled witch hazel on a cotton ball (this may sting) (also see *Homeopathy* section).
- Apply comfrey leaf, yarrow, yellow dock root or mullein ointment or poultices externally to reduce swelling, ease pain, and stop bleeding.
- Sit fifteen to thirty minutes in a shallow bath containing one-pint/500 millilitres of witch hazel infusion or one-pint/500 millilitres each of comfrey leaf and echinacea tea. Or try sitting in a sitz bath with Epsom salts to bring relief.

Swelling of Legs, Ankles, and Feet

- Avoid excessive salt intake.
- Make sure your water/fluid intake is adequate.
- Try the remedies for varicosities (also see *Homeopathy* section).
- Elevate the feet whenever possible. Use a padded footrest to prop the feet up.
- Do not dangle feet or cross legs at the knee.
- Avoid constricting clothing and shoes.
- Use gel shoe inserts or orthotics to take the pressure off the feet.
- Get regular exercise (e.g. a brisk daily walk or swim, pre-natal yoga).
- Have an Epson salt foot soak nightly and have your partner gently massage your feet (working the fluid towards the heart).

Note: If the swelling is in your legs or feet swelling is severe, accompanied by headaches and/or an increase in blood pressure, contact your health care practitioner *immediately* as it may be a sign of toxaemia.

Note: If you experience carpal tunnel symptoms (tingling in fingers, wrist weakness and/or pain) during pregnancy, it may also be due to water retention. Follow the same dietary and herbal advice as for foot swelling and varicosities and make sure to be checked by your chiropractor for nerve root involvement (see *Chart of Effects of Spinal Misalignments*).

Leg and Foot Cramps

- Can be caused by malabsorption of calcium, disturbance of the calcium-magnesium-phosphorus ratio, pressure from the pregnant uterus on blood vessels and/or varicosities. (See the *Table of Herbs That Contain Calcium*).
- Get regular exercise.
- Try chiropractic and/or light massage (deep massage can sometimes cause a painful bruise and will not bring relief) (See *Chiropractic* section and *Chart of Effects of Spinal Misalignments* for more information).
- Use gel insoles or orthotics in your shoes for extra cushioning and support.
- Try the remedies for varicosities, especially vitamin E.
- Stretch the affected calf by pointing the heel of the foot (not the toe). Hold for a few seconds, and then relax your leg completely. Repeat as often as necessary.

- When experiencing a cramp in the foot, extend the leg by pointing the heel.
- If you get frequent foot cramps, strengthen the muscles in the arch by placing a towel flat on the floor in front of you. Sit on chair, remove your shoes and socks, and place your heel on the towel. Use your toes to scrunch and wrinkle the towel towards you. Do this exercise two times per foot, twice a day at first then gradually work up to five repetitions, twice a day. Go very gently at first so that you don't cause foot cramps from over-exertion.

Slowing Down of the Digestive Tract

(e.g. constipation, hard, or infrequent stools)

- Avoid commercial iron supplements, excess bread, dairy products and red meat.
- Increase your fluid intake (six to eight glasses of water daily plus soup and juices).
- Get regular exercise.
- Eat two apples per day, lots of raw vegetables, whole grains, prunes, fresh greens and supplement with bulk fibre if necessary (e.g. ground flax or psyllium).
- Take a mild bitter such as dandelion leaf or chamomile.

Gas

- Try ginger, fennel seed, dill, peppermint leaves, and/or chamomile tea.

Bleeding or Puffy Gums

- Frequently due to the hormonal changes associated with pregnancy.
- Switch to an extra soft toothbrush.
- Make sure to brush and floss your teeth gently at least twice a day.
- See your dentist for a check-up at least once during your pregnancy.
- Make sure you are taking in enough vitamin C, B-group vitamins and protein to promote healing of the gums.

Nausea/Vomiting/Morning Sickness

- Eat frequent small meals (e.g. dry toast or unsalted crackers before getting out of bed) and protein-rich snacks.
- Get regular exercise.
- Drink plenty of water (six to eight glasses per day).

- Try wearing a motion-sickness band (known as a "sea band").
- Don't take your pre-natal vitamin until later in the day as the iron in it may be contributing to your nausea.
- Increase your B-group vitamins, especially vitamin B6 (found in wheat germ, wheat bran, beef liver, cod, turkey, beef, banana, brussels sprouts, cabbage and mango).
- Increase your vitamin K (found in nettle leaves, alfalfa, broccoli, brussels sprouts, green cabbage, kelp, natural yogurt, egg yolk, safflower oil, and fish liver oil) and vitamin C.
- Use red raspberry leaf, peppermint leaf or spearmint leaf, ginger, lemon balm, chamomile and/or peach leaf teas.
- Also see *Homeopathy* section.

Heartburn

- Try eating a more carbohydrate-based meal (e.g. rice, beans, pasta) before bedtime.
- Eat smaller, more frequent meals.
- Stay upright for a one to two hours after eating.
- Drink ginger tea (put half a teaspoon of fresh grated ginger in a cup of boiling water. Let steep for ten minutes then strain out the ginger. Cool to a drinkable temperature and drink).
- Try slippery elm bark tea.
- Try eating natural/raw almonds or natural yogurt.
- Drinking a cold glass of milk may also help (personally, I found eating a few spoonfuls of all natural chocolate ice cream to be more helpful for soothing heartburn).
- Try chewable papaya enzyme tablets.
- Sometimes chewing natural spearmint or peppermint-flavoured gum helps.
- Also try drinking anise, fennel, or dill seed tea (two teaspoons of seeds to one cup boiling water. Cover and let steep five to ten minutes, then strain and drink a few teaspoons every few minutes).
- Also see *Homeopathy* section.
- Try a specific chiropractic adjustment for a pseudo-hiatus hernia (see *Chiropractic* section and *Chart of Effects of Spinal Misalignments* for more information).
- Press on the acupressure point located in the web between your thumb and first finger of your *left* hand. It is usually tender and is easily pressed using a pincer grasp of your thumb and first finger of the right hand. Avoid working the same spot on your right hand as it may increase your risk of miscarriage.

- If none of the above works, use a natural calcium-based antacid (available in most health food stores) as needed for relief. Avoid antacids containing magnesium or aluminium salts and artificial sweeteners as they may harm the baby.

Low Spirits

- Improve digestion (see previous *Slowing Down of the Digestive Tract* section), avoid constipation and low blood sugar levels.
- Get regular exercise.
- Treat yourself to a regular facial, manicure and/or pedicure.
- Post pictures of beautiful babies, utilize visualization and do something special to commemorate your pregnancy such as pregnancy photos, a belly cast, etc.
- Keep a special journal of your pregnancy experience.
- Talk, read and sing to your baby.
- Get support by talking to other expectant parents or a trusted friend.
- Use birthing affirmations daily (*Appendix One*) and create your birth plan.
- Try meditation, yoga, Hypnobirthing®, listening to inspiring music, and/or reading a great parenting book (see *Pre-natal Yoga*).
- Try supplementing with cod liver oil (in the winter months) or fish oil (in the summer months).
- Try dandelion root bitters, dandelion leaf, chamomile, burdock root, chicory root, spearmint, and/or peppermint teas.
- Also see *Homeopathy* section.

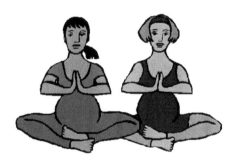

Worry, Anxiety and Tension

- Use calming herbs such as chamomile, skullcap, valerian root, passionflower, lemon balm and motherwort (also see *Homeopathy* section).
- Get regular exercise such as going for a brisk, daily walk, or swimming.

- Arm yourself with information and support by attending a pre-natal or childbirth education class, going on a hospital/birth facility tour, and/or talking to other expectant parents or a trusted friend.
- Try meditation, yoga, Tai Chi, daily birthing affirmations, visualization, Hypnobirthing® and/or breath work.

Mental Fogginess

(Also known as 'Pregnancy Brain' or 'Mommy Brain').

- Try to take regular naps.
- Write a short 'To Do' list of three to four things that need to be done and delegate the rest to your partner, friends or family.
- Place important items (e.g. keys, purse) in the same special spot each time.
- Get regular gentle exercise to increase circulation.
- Remember to have a sense of humour!
- Try craniosacral therapy, meditation, visualization, and/or yoga.

Group B Streptococcus

(Confirmed by a positive vaginal/rectal swab or urine sample).

- Supplement with vitamin C and eat a *lot* of fresh garlic every day.
- At thirty-two weeks, start drinking one cup of burdock root and echinacea root infusion daily (made by steeping one-half ounce/fifteen grams of each of these herbs in four cups/one litre of boiling water for two hours; strain and store the rest in the refrigerator).
- Take one-half teaspoon each of echinacea and astragalus tinctures twice daily.
- Eat a diet rich in probiotics, e.g. natural yogurt with active cultures and fermented vegetables (e.g. sauerkraut, pickles, miso, tempeh, etc.) or take a probiotic supplement.

Labour Helpers

- Use red raspberry leaf tea to prepare the uterus beforehand.
- To initiate labour, use blue cohosh or a combination of blue cohosh, black cohosh, partridgeberry, red raspberry leaf and cinnamon.
- Also see *Homeopathy* section for more specific labour helpers.
- To initiate labour, try castor oil rubbed on the abdomen or taken internally (one part castor oil mixed with two or more parts orange juice

and two parts vodka or other alcohol). Castor oil taken internally is not recommended unless you are *very* determined to initiate labour as it will likely cause very uncomfortable intestinal cramping and possibly diarrhoea.

- Take a hot bath, eat a spicy meal, and/or go for a long, brisk walk/hike.
- Relax and focus on daily activities instead of dwelling on labour.
- Make love, have an orgasm or try nipple stimulation (a particularly effective technique is having your partner use the back of his/her fingertips/nails to stroke in the direction of the armpit towards the nipples).
- Try a specific labour-starter chiropractic adjustment. Additionally, adjustments during labour can ease discomfort and help to move things along if they have slowed or stalled (see *Chiropractic* section and *Chart of Effects of Spinal Misalignments* for more information).
- Try acupressure: Spleen 6 is located approximately three fingers width above the inside ankle bone, under the ridge of the shin bone. Once located (the mother will let you know you're one the right spot!), press both legs with your thumbs, hold for ten seconds then release. Repeat a total of three times. The reflex points for the ovaries and uterus are located under the ankle bones in the centre of the heel on both sides of the foot (medial and lateral). Squeeze them together, both feet at the same time, using thumbs and middle fingers. Hold for ten seconds and release. Repeat a total of three times. There are also many acupressure points in the lower back/sacral area that can ease labour and back pains. Additionally, stimulating the toenail on the pinkie toe with light scratching can help ease labour pains as well as move the labour forward.
- Use visualization (see *Appendix Two* for a rose (cervix) opening visualization that can be helpful), birth affirmations, meditation, Hypnobirthing®, hydrotherapy (tub or shower) and/or progressive relaxation to relax and release any fears.
- For exhaustion during labour, use ginseng or ginger to send energy to the womb.
- For prolonged labour, try stimulating the reflex points in the hands by holding a strong plastic or metal comb in each hand so that your fingertips support the edge and your palms receive the pressure from the teeth of the combs. Press the combs into your palms with each contraction.
- See also *Fifty Comfort Measures to Ease Labour Discomfort*.

Returning the Uterus, Perineum and Abdominal Muscles to Normal More Quickly

- Prevent tearing by practising perineal massage from thirty-five weeks onwards. Use slightly warmed olive, almond, or other natural oil and have your partner use their thumb or two fingers (or use your own) to gently massage and stretch the perineal area. Work in a "U" pattern from front to back, carefully avoiding the urethral area (the very front). Only stretch the vaginal walls until a *light* burning sensation is felt. And always make sure hands are clean and fingernails are neatly trimmed before starting!
- Do *lots* of Kegel exercises (before and after the birth) to tighten the muscles around your vagina and anus. From day one after the birth, try to do Kegels every time you feed your baby so it is easier to remember. To isolate these muscles, imagine you are trying to stop yourself from passing urine. Hold the contraction of these muscles as long as you are able, remembering to breathe, and then relax. Repeat the exercise up to ten repetitions each time, two to three times a day.
- Once the above Kegel exercises become easy, try adding "Super Kegels." Tighten inside as if you are trying to stop yourself from passing urine—HOLD. As you feel the tightening feeling starting to fade, tighten again and HOLD. Repeat tightening and HOLD five seconds, then relax. Repeat five times. Remember to breathe!
- Use breastfeeding and gentle exercise.
- Red raspberry leaf, vitex, lemon balm, hawthorne and/or fennel tea can be helpful.
- See *Homeopathy* section—Arnica Montana is especially helpful post-partum.
- Use the squirt bottle ("irri-bottle") provided by the hospital to pour warm water on your perineum while you're going to the bathroom. The water dilutes your urine so it doesn't sting as much when it comes in contact with your skin. Cleanse yourself with another squirt afterward.
- Expose the wound to air as much as possible.
- Use a comfrey leaf sitz bath: a soothing solution that speeds healing of the perineum post-partum can be made from the leaves steeped in hot water, and added to a warm bath. Do not use on dirty wounds as the rapid healing can trap the dirt or pus. A sitz bath is a shallow plastic basin that you fill with warm water and position over your toilet seat. It makes it convenient to soak your bottom several times a day without having to fill a tub full of water and completely undress each time.

- Sitting in a tub of clean, warm water several times a day will feel good to your perineum, whether the discomfort is due to stitches or bruising from the birth.
- Ice packs and witch hazel compresses can be soothing.
- Do *not* use aspirin or ibuprofen while breastfeeding. If your doctor or midwife recommends taking acetaminophen (e.g. Tylenol) or other pain reliever with codeine, watch closely for signs of toxicity in the baby (e.g. excessive sleepiness, unresponsiveness, slowed breathing, jaundice). Some women's bodies convert codeine into significant amounts of morphine, which can pose serious problems for the infant.
- Sit with your legs together, but not crossed. Try not to sit too long at a time.
- Do gentle pelvic tilts to start to re-tighten the abdominal muscles from day one after the birth. Lie on your back with your knees bent. As you continue to breathe normally, tighten your abdominal muscles to flatten your back against the bed. Hold this position for five seconds then relax your muscles and feel the natural lower back curve return. Repeat ten times.

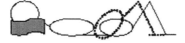

This exercise can also be done standing against a wall but remember to use good posture: keep your chin tucked in and shoulders relaxed against the wall.

- From day two onwards, you can lie on your stomach with a pillow under your hips and also under your shoulders (to relieve pressure on your breasts and maintain good neck posture) for up to twenty minutes a day to help relieve after pains and to help your uterus shrink and return to its natural position.

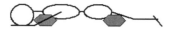

- Before doing the following abdominal exercises, check your abdominal muscles by doing a pelvic tilt with your knees bent and using one hand to feel the middle of your abdomen for a gap or bulge in the abdominal muscles. If there is a bulge or gap wider than two finger widths, do the first exercise only. If there is no bulge or the gap is two fingers wide or less, do all four exercises. The key to these exercises is to maintain the pelvic tilt.

◊   Knee Raise—lying with your hands under your lower back, pelvic tilt to keep your back flat, and slowly bring your right knee towards your chest. Hold five to ten seconds while exhaling. Slowly return to the starting position while inhaling and repeat with your left knee. Repeat ten times each side.

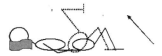

◊   Leg Extension—lying with your hands under your lower back, pelvic tilt to keep your back flat. Slowly bend and then straighten your right leg, keeping it approximately two inches off the bed/floor while slowly exhaling. Inhale, bend the knee and return the leg to its starting position (foot on the floor, knee bent). Do the same with your left leg and repeat five times each side.

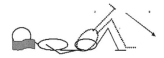

◊   Curl-Up—lying with your hands by your sides, do a pelvic tilt, tuck your chin in slightly, stare at a spot on the ceiling and raise your head off the bed/floor while breathing out. Hold for five seconds then slowly relax back. Repeat five to ten times. When you are able to do this easily ten times, then progress to raising your head and shoulders off the bed/floor.

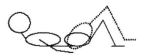

◊   Diagonal Curl-Up—Repeat as per the curl-up above but reach with your right hand towards your left knee and then with your left hand to your right knee while breathing out. Repeat five to ten times each side.

Breast Sensitivity, Swelling, and Engorgement

- Use external cold cabbage leaf or potato poultices.
- Alternate using cool compresses (not cold) and warm compresses.
- Warm showers are also useful to relieve the discomfort associated with engorgement.
- Take one teaspoon of echinacea tincture daily.
- Also see *Homeopathy* section.
- Wear a non-constricting bra (non-compressive sports bra or try a tank top with a shelf bra). Avoid underwire bras
- Breast massage can also help: use warm massage oil or cream and make large circles around the outside of each breast (individually or both at the same time), avoiding the nipple or areola. Do this for several minutes. Then massage one breast at a time, using the fingertips to make small circles around each breast. After several minutes, repeat on the other breast. Lastly, place both hands flat on either side of the areola, with the thumbs pointing towards your head and the fingers pointing towards your waist. Then slowly slide your hands away from the areola until you reach the edge of the breast. Be sure to avoid direct massage on the sensitive areola region. Turn your hand slightly to cover a different portion of the breast and repeat. Do this for one or two minutes then massage the other breast.
- Soften breasts by expressing or pumping some milk.
- Nurse baby often!

Sore Nipples

- Avoid constricting clothing. Avoid plastic against the nipples.
- Use only plain water for washing.
- Use rough towels and self-massage to toughen the skin.
- Make sure baby is latching correctly (see *Sucking Problems*).
- Break suction with your baby finger before taking baby off the breast.
- Offer the least sore breast first.
- Squeeze some of your breast milk onto the nipples then air-dry nipples.
- Apply comfrey, plantain or calendula salves to soothe (wash off before breastfeeding).
- Pure lanolin cream is also soothing to the skin of the nipples and breasts and promotes speedy healing.
- Also see *Homeopathy* section.

Breastfeeding Problems

- First, always make sure that the baby is latching correctly. If uncertain, check with your doctor or midwife, a lactation consultant or support group such as the La Leche League for more information (see *Reference and Resources* section, *Sucking Problems*, and also *New Baby Ergonomics—Tips To Prevent The Aches And Pains That Can Come with Becoming a New Parent*).
- Have the sucking and rooting reflexes checked by your doctor, midwife or chiropractor. (See also *Sucking Problems*).
- An article in the March 2007 Journal of Clinical Chiropractic Paediatrics presented three documented case studies of chiropractic care helping new mothers to produce more milk. The researchers concluded that subluxations and the neurological interference that they cause can play a major role in hypolactation (a reduction in the production of mother's milk). (See also *Chiropractic* section or http://www.icpa4kids.org/research/chiropractic/breastfeeding.htm).
- Consider using a breast pump to ensure the breasts are completely emptied each time and also to increase the frequency of stimulation to help increase milk supply.
- Make sure you are taking in enough fluids (e.g. minimum eight glasses of water per day), adequate calories (similar to the *Basic Pregnancy Diet*), and in particular, eating plenty of protein. Breastfeeding is *not* a time to diet!
- Avoid constricting bras and clothing.
- Signs your baby is breastfeeding well in the first three weeks are:

  ◊ has four to eight noticeably wet diapers in a twenty-four hour period by three or four days of age (usually the urine is pale and odourless);
  ◊ has at least two to five bowel movements in a twenty-four hour period (progressing from brownish to seedy mustard yellow-coloured, and at least the size of a loonie or silver dollar);
  ◊ breastfeeds *at least* eight times (ideally ten to twelve times) in twenty-four hours;
  ◊ is content after most feedings;
  ◊ you can hear your baby swallowing during feedings;
  ◊ breastfeeding doesn't hurt;
  ◊ your breasts are full before feedings and soft after feedings; and
  ◊ your baby is drinking only breast milk.

- Also see *Homeopathy* section.

Blessed Thistle (Cnicus benedictus)

Blessed thistle is famed for its ability to increase and enrich breast milk supply, especially when used with red raspberry leaf and/or fenugreek. It is also said to remove suicidal feelings and lift depression. Commonly taken as a tincture: ten to twenty drops (two millilitres) two to four times per day. Stimulates appetite and can be used to help with female reproductive problems. Blessed thistle has a laxative and emetic (causes vomiting) effect in large doses—do *not* use during pregnancy.

Fenugreek (Trigonella foenum-graecum)

Fenugreek seed has been used to increase milk production since biblical times.

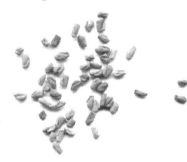

The herb contains phytoestrogens, which are plant chemicals similar to the female sex hormone estrogen. Fenugreek seeds contain hormone precursors that increase milk supply. Some believe this is because breasts are modified sweat glands, and fenugreek stimulates sweat production. It has been found that fenugreek can increase a nursing mother's milk supply within twenty-four to seventy-two hours after first taking the herb. Once an adequate level of milk production is reached, most women can discontinue the fenugreek and maintain the milk supply with adequate breast stimulation. Fenugreek can be taken in tea form, although tea is believed to be less potent than the pills and the tea comes with a bitter taste that can be hard to stomach. Fenugreek is not right for everyone: the herb has caused aggravated asthma symptoms in some women and has lowered blood glucose levels in some women with diabetes. Fenugreek seed can cause uterine contractions—do *not* use if you're pregnant.

Borage Leaf (Borago officinalis)

Borage leaves insure an abundant supply of milk, act as a mild laxative and soothe jangled nerves. This ancient herb is associated with courage and in medieval times was infused in wine as a tonic to banish melancholy. Even today, an infusion of borage leaves is nature's best tonic for stress and stress related problems. The leaves contain vitamin C and are rich in calcium, potassium and mineral salts. European herbalists use borage tea to restore strength during convalescence. The leaves are used as an adrenal tonic to balance and restore the health of the adrenal glands following periods of stress. It is of particular benefit during recovery from surgery or following steroid treatment. An *infusion* of borage acts as a galactogogue, promoting the production of milk in breastfeeding mothers. Tea made from the leaves and flowers can also relieve fevers, and promote sweating. To make an infusion, pour one cup of boiling water over a quarter of a cup of bruised fresh leaves. Steep for five minutes, strain, and drink.

Note: Borage grows very commonly as a weed in West Coast gardens. It has large, slightly 'furry' leaves and small blue-purple clusters of flowers.

Fennel/Barley Water (Foeniculum vulgare/Hordeum vulgare)

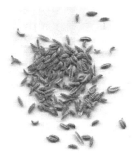

This combination not only increases the breast milk but eases after pains and settles the digestion of mom and baby. Prepare barley water by soaking half a cup pearled (regular) barley in three cups water overnight or by boiling for twenty-five minutes. Strain out barley and discard it (or add it to soup). Heat a cup or two of the barley water to boiling as needed (refrigerate the remaining barley water) and pour over one teaspoon of fennel seeds and steep no longer than thirty minutes.

Hops Flowers (Humulus lupulus)

Hops flowers bring sleep along with increased breast milk flow. Beer is a convenient source of hops but beware of domestic brands that may contain potentially harmful chemicals and preservatives. Look for organic or imported beers that are additive-free; alcohol and chemical-free brews of hops and malt are also available in some health food stores.

General Note: Most of the time teas, especially those containing caffeine, should be avoided during lactation, unless used for a specific medicinal purpose. A list of herbal teas considered safe in moderation (no more than two to three cups of tea per day) include: red raspberry leaf, blackberry leaf, citrus peel, ginger, lemon balm, mint, rose hip, linden flower (not recommended for those who have heart problems) and strawberry leaf.

Dr. Stacey Rosenberg

Nursing Formula

Stimulates milk production and flow and restores vitality to weary mothers. It can also restore tone to the mother's digestive system and can help with colic and indigestion in the baby.

One-ounce/thirty grams dried blessed thistle or borage leaves
One-ounce/thirty grams dried red raspberry or nettle leaves
One-teaspoon/five grams of any one of these seeds:
fenugreek, fennel, caraway, anise, cumin, or coriander.

Place leaves in a half-gallon/two litre jar and fill to the top with boiling water. Cap tightly and let steep overnight. Strain out herbs and refrigerate the infusion until needed. As you get ready to nurse, pour out one cupful of the brew and heat it to nearly boiling. Pour it over a teaspoon of the seeds, let it steep (a bodum or coffee plunger pot works really well for this) and then cool five more minutes before drinking. This brew can be drunk freely, up to two quarts/two litres daily, if desired.

Sucking Problems

- If you have concerns with your newborn's ability to nurse, such as pain when nursing, cracked or sore nipples, having to use awkward or two different holds (e.g. one breast is a cradle hold, one breast is a football hold) to help baby latch, baby's not gaining weight or not content/satisfied after feedings, have the baby's suck evaluated by your doctor, midwife or Doctor of Chiropractic.
- Other signs to watch for that indicate your baby may need an adjustment to assist with sucking include: baby won't open its mouth wide enough to effectively latch, baby's mouth opens asymmetrically (especially easy to see when baby cries—check if mouth opens wider on one side), and if baby had a fast or difficult delivery (especially if interventions such as vacuum suction or forceps were used) particularly if there is a lot of cranial bone moulding.
- Sucking is a reflex, but it is also a co-ordinated muscular action. An effective suck cycle involves co-ordination of jaw motion with peri-oral muscles and tongue movement, adequate changes in sucking pressure, and peristaltic tongue movement.
- Sucking dysfunction is the most common and often the only sign of a neurological disorder. The rooting reflex should always be checked first, sucking reflex, then the quality of the suck, then the cranial nerves (see *Chiropractic* section).

- You can help baby latch better by:

  ◊ Get comfortable (use pillows as necessary) (see also *New Baby Ergonomics—Tips To Prevent The Aches And Pains That Can Come with Becoming a New Parent section*);
  ◊ Hold baby facing you with her tummy against you;
  ◊ Baby's nose should be at the level of the nipple with her head slightly tilted back;
  ◊ Put your hand further under your breast, placing your fingers close to your chest (cross-cradle hold);
  ◊ Wait until baby opens her mouth as wide as a yawn; and
  ◊ Bring baby close. More of the areola should be showing above her upper lip than below her lower lip (aim your nipple towards the roof of her mouth).
  ◊ If she is on well, you should see her mouth open at a wide angle and you should be comfortable with baby nursing actively (and no nipple discomfort!).

Crying

- Babies universally cry as a way to promote contact with the mother: to convey nutritional needs, to communicate pain, to release current tension or to release tension from past trauma.
- There are two main reasons that babies cry: to communicate a need or discomfort (e.g. hungry, cold, wet, bored, or just wanting to be held) and 'irritable crying' where all their physical needs have been met and it is more likely to be an emotional reason for the crying (e.g. frustration, confusion, fear, over stimulation, birth trauma may be stored in the body as emotional pain or tension that needs to be released through crying).
- The quality of the cry may indicate the problem: a louder, more persistent cry may indicate pain; a less intense, frequent cry may indicate inadequate parental responsiveness.
- A baby should *never* be left to cry alone!
- There are many ways to soothe a crying baby without using a pacifier:

  ◊ Breastfeeding—use your breast as a pacifier and provide skin-to-skin contact. Introducing a pacifier too early may cause nipple confusion, as breastfeeding requires different muscle action and tongue position than sucking on a pacifier.

Note: A breastfed baby who is not gaining weight should *never* be given a pacifier.

- ◊ Swaddling—wrapping up baby can work though it may take longer to calm him. Make sure baby is not overheating (check for sweating or moisture on the back of the neck);
- ◊ Singing—your voice has a calming effect on baby;
- ◊ Rocking—the rhythm of a rocking chair can be calming;
- ◊ Walking—go for a walk with baby;
- ◊ Bathing—try taking a warm bath with your baby; and/or
- ◊ Try to maintain a consistent routine, especially around bedtime or fussy periods.

- To the parent, inconsolable crying is colic.

Colic

- Symptoms of colic include: relentless crying, restless sleep, abdominal pain, baby's legs are flexed, and there may be abdominal problems secondary to vagus nerve irritation.
- Colic affects twenty-five to thirty-five percent of all infants especially if an elder sibling had colic, there were pregnancy complications (in particular, maternal depression, maternal medication, forceps delivery, epidural anaesthesia, and/or Pitocin use), and is more common with educated parents.
- Colic is extremely stressful for the family. Mothers of babies with colic are more likely to be depressed than other mothers. Some parents cannot cope and respond with aggression. Make sure you seek help from your doctor/midwife or chiropractor before it affects you in this way.
- The colicky baby should have normal growth and development (healthy baby, worried parents).
- Colic is not due to an immature digestive tract, increased wind in the digestive tract, cow's milk allergy, anxious new parents, poor sleep regulation or sleep disorders.
- Literature reviews have found that the following treatments for colic do *not* work:

- ◊ Antacids, analgesics, prostaglandins, progesterone, formula change, change from breast milk to formula, feeding upright, vertical position, herbal teas, alcohol, homatropine, phenobarbitone, vestibular stimulation, holding, moving car or swing, counselling, parent retraining, quitting smoking, nipple change, pacifier use, antispasmodics, antihistamines, simethicone, gripe water, baking soda, apple cider vinegar socks, letting baby cry it out, white noise (e.g. hairdryer or vacuum cleaner), heart beat tape, or midwife hold.

- The only medical treatment that 'works' is dicyclomine hydrochloride (babies stopped crying in sixty-three percent of cases) but the side effects include apnoea (breathing stops), collapse, seizures, coma and death. This is *not* a safe treatment and should *never* be used.
- Several chiropractic studies have found that anywhere between seventy and ninety-four percent of colicky infants improved with chiropractic care, usually within three treatments.

Gastro-Esophageal Reflux

- This condition is heralded by colicky symptoms with normal post-feeding vomiting and seemingly effortless "spitting up" which can go on for quite some time after feeding is complete. Normally, there is no abdominal bloating.
- The vomiting may be projectile. If there is a fever accompanying the projectile vomiting, see your health care provider immediately.
- This condition responds well to chiropractic treatment (see *Chart of Effects of Spinal Misalignments*).
- Fennel/barley water may also help.
- Occasionally, antacids are needed to limit the vomiting and to protect the baby's oesophagus from acid erosions. See your health care provider.

Cow's Milk Protein Intolerance

- Occurs in approximately seven percent of the entire infant population.
- Not limited to formula-fed babies, breast-fed babies may also have cow's milk protein intolerance if mom is drinking milk or eating dairy.
- Usually starts around thirteen weeks of age.
- Babies have respiratory, skin, and gastro-intestinal signs and symptoms:

  ◊ Excess mucus production, 'rattley' bronchial sounds, recurrent upper respiratory tract infections, and/or chronic cough (see also *Homeopathy* section);
  ◊ Fine skin rash—particularly in and around the buttocks, creases of the body, hair line and trunk; eczema; excoriations in the peri-anal area, and/or signs of thrush (Candida infection) in the vulva and peri-anal areas; and
  ◊ Constipation, diarrhoea or alternating constipation/diarrhoea; mild regurgitating and/or vomiting; bloating due to gaseous distension of the bowels; excessive flatulence and burping.

- Treatment involves mother giving up dairy for at least three weeks and then re-assessing the child for breast-fed infants or switching to a pre-digested formula (e.g. Nutramagen) or soy based formula for formula-fed babies.
- Approximately sixty-seven percent of babies who are cow's milk intolerant are also intolerant to soy-based formulas. There may be an initial improvement once switched to soy, which is not sustained once the immune system develops antibodies to the new protein.
- Goat's milk may also be used but must be supplemented as it is deficient in folic acid and vitamin B12 (see *Appendix Four—Infant Formula Fortification Protocol*).

Irritable Infant Syndrome (Musculoskeletal Origin)

- Characterised by: excessive crying, arching posture (leaning back or arching up when baby is placed on its tummy), hypertonia (very tight muscles), limb hyperactivity, sensitivity to touch, restless sleep, unusual posture at rest (e.g. prefers not to lie on its back), general unrest, and/or appetite or eating problems.
- Chiropractic care has been shown as safe and efficacious therapy for IISMO as well as colic (see *Babies and Chiropractic: A Parent's Guide*).

Note: The half-life (the amount of time for half of a substance to be eliminated from the body) of caffeine in a newborn's body is seventy to eighty hours, compared to six hours in an adult. So make sure to strictly limit or eliminate your caffeine intake while breastfeeding until your baby is at least three to six months old. After three months of age, they begin to develop the enzymes needed to process and eliminate caffeine more efficiently from their system.

Birth Trauma

- Can occur even in a "normal" birth but is more common with assisted births (e.g. forceps or vacuum extraction). Elective caesarean deliveries can also result in injury to the baby, but it is more common in emergency c-sections where the baby has descended into the birth canal.
- Risk factors include: intrauterine misalignment, use of extraction aids, prolonged labour and multiple foetuses.
- Mild to moderate soft tissue injuries are common in birth and it is thought that many musculoskeletal complaints that are common throughout life begin at birth (see *Chiropractic and Babies* and *Chiropractic: A Parent's Guide* sections).

- "When it comes to obstetric accidents, it is interesting to know that although obstetricians make up only three per cent of all medical doctors, they account for twenty-nine per cent of all the costs and damages, and account for thirty per cent of all claims of negligence against medical doctors! This means that one-third of all mistakes made by doctors are made by those responsible for delivering our children!" A 1993 review of literature by Marc Gottlieb determined that despite these statistics "birth trauma still remains an under-publicized and, therefore, under-treated problem. And when it comes to trauma from the birth process, we are generally talking about damage to the skull, spinal column, and brachial areas." (French R, 2002).
- Suboccipital strain (KISS Syndrome), torticollis (wry neck), spinal joint dysfunction, cranial distortions, excessive moulding of the cranial bones, incessant crying, feeding difficulties, head banging or pulling, lowered resistance to illness are all signs of birth trauma and respond well to gentle chiropractic care.

Newborn Jaundice

- About fifty to sixty percent of full-term babies have a yellowish cast to their skin during their first week or two of life. For most babies, this is a temporary, harmless condition that will go away on its own or with mild treatment.
- Jaundice quite often begins two to three days after birth and is usually gone by day ten or fourteen.
- Always talk to your midwife or doctor if you notice that your baby has jaundice.
- Quite often responds to daily exposure of sunlight. Often ten minutes a day in the summer is enough to clear the jaundice within a week. Be sure to cover baby's eyes. In the winter months, special lights may be necessary.
- Make sure baby is getting enough breast milk, as insufficient fluids can make it harder for him to eliminate the excess bilirubin. Try to breastfeed ten to twelve times a day. Water supplementation does not help reduce the serum bilirubin.

13

Chiropractic

When D.D. Palmer gave that first adjustment to Harvey Lillard in 1895, he could not know how far reaching his theory and his understanding would reach!

At first he thought it was a cure for deafness as Harvey Lillard's hearing was restored by that first adjustment. Then as he adjusted many deaf people, some who had their hearing restored and some who did not, he discovered that chiropractic actually enhanced an individual's overall health as well as noticing that conditions and symptoms were improved.

What is Chiropractic?

Chiropractic grew from an adjustment that restored Harvey Lillard's hearing to become a science, philosophy and art that is focused on the correction and prevention of subluxation to enhance human potential. Subluxation is a disease that interferes with the expression of innate intelligence and the function of the nervous system, which controls all organs and tissues in the human body.

How Does Chiropractic Work?

A person's spine is made of twenty-four moveable bones called vertebrae, plus the sacrum (tailbone), pelvis, and skull.

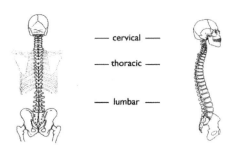

From the brain, nerve impulses travel down the spinal cord and branch out into nerves, exiting between the vertebrae. When the vertebrae become misaligned or unable to move properly, it irritates and interferes with the nerves. This is called a subluxation. The message from the brain is slowed down and the life energy carried by the nerve is unable to reach the organs and tissues at one hundred per cent of its potential (see *Chart of Effects of Spinal Misalignments* section).

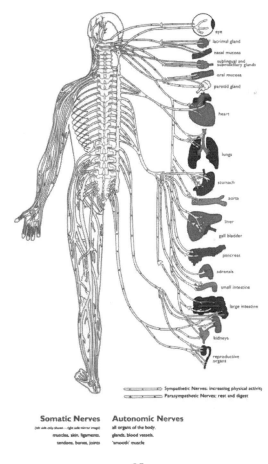

95

Your nervous system controls, coordinates, and gives life to all the cells of your body. It also senses all of your cells and integrates your emotions and conscious thoughts.

A Chiropractor aligns the vertebrae through gentle adjustments to the spine, relieving the pressure on the nerves and allowing one hundred per cent of the nerve energy to reach the tissues it serves. Chiropractic care is natural, simply removing interference to your body's own controlling and healing ability, called innate intelligence. A Doctor of Chiropractic's primary goal is to assist your amazing, internal healing wisdom by removing interference to your nervous system called subluxations.

Spinal Dysfunction

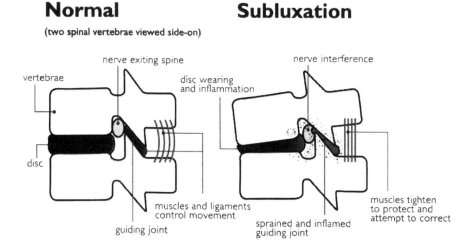

As your pregnancy advances, some Chiropractic techniques will need to be modified for your comfort. Your Chiropractor is aware of this and will make the necessary changes. In particular, special pregnancy pillows or chiropractic benches with drop-away abdominal sections are used to accommodate your growing belly. Side-lying lower back or pelvis adjustments should be avoided, especially in the second and third trimester due to discomfort, ligamentous laxity, and a small risk of placental abruption.

How Does Subluxation Occur?

The first misalignments in the spine often occur during the birth process. A 'normal' birth can put upwards of forty pounds of pressure through the baby's fragile head and neck. And if the doctor assists, studies have shown that up to 120 pounds of pressure and traction can be used (especially in the case of forceps or vacuum extraction)! Learning to walk, ride a bike, climb a tree, and all the jolts, slips, bumps, and falls that go with most childhood activities are major causes of subluxations. Sports, auto accidents, repetitive motion, work injuries, chills, and poor posture are other physical causes of subluxations. Pregnancy weight gain, changes in posture and gait and hormonal changes all can cause subluxations. The way we walk, stand, sit, and sleep is affected by and directly impacts the functioning of the spine! In addition, certain foods, drugs, alcohol, allergens, and other chemical substances may react with your body and create subluxations. Dehydration is also a key cause of spinal dysfunction. As well, emotional stress and negativity can affect the functioning of your spine through the tension that it causes. In short, subluxations occur when your body receives a physical, biochemical, or emotional stress that it cannot adapt to.

How Long Will It Take To Heal?

Your spine has many segments that contribute to movement and has the ability to compensate for small regions that are not moving correctly. Because of this, you can have many subluxations that can exist for years without you being aware of them. As each successive subluxation is formed, your spine and nervous system becomes less flexible, making the effects of each new subluxation cumulative. It is only when your spine cannot compensate any further (or during an excessive stress) that malfunctioning segments are forced to move which causes inflammation in the local tissues and splinting in the supporting muscles and then pain begins. Like tooth decay (cavities), you often don't feel any obvious symptoms until subluxations have been developing for some time.

Studies have shown that it only takes as little as 10mm of mercury pressure (approximately the weight of a dime) to alter the nerve root and dorsal root ganglion's ability to function normally. These alterations would therefore alter the quality and/or quantity of the message sent. At the tissue and cellular level, the message received would not be adequate for the function the body demands. The entire body could then theoretically be affected.

The longer a spinal problem has been present, the longer it takes to correct. The muscles and ligaments have become accustomed to the incorrect positioning and movement of the vertebrae. In addition, many patients do not seek chiropractic care until symptoms occur. For that reason, it may take a series of adjustments before the muscles become used to holding the vertebrae in the proper position, allowing for full nerve function. It takes retraining of these structures to overcome this 'memory pattern' of the tissues surrounding the spine. If subluxations are left uncorrected, spinal decay (formerly called osteoarthritis) may be the result. Chiropractic is about restoring the function of the nervous system, not covering up symptoms!

Spinal Decay

Normal	Phase 1	Phase 2	Phase 3
Disc spaces appear healthy.	Loss of normal curves and alignment.	Disc has worn considerably.	Spinal segment has fused completely, nerve openings are greatly narrowed.
Alignment is normal.	Supporting tissues weakened.	To compensate, the body has begun to stiffen itself with calcium.	Adjacent segments will wear more quickly under the extra stress.
No degeneration is evident.	Abnormal movement irritates nerves and other tissues.	Continued nerve irritation is present.	

You Choose Your Level of Benefit From Chiropractic

Basic or Initial Intensive Care

This level of care is designed to stabilize your spine and begin to improve its function as soon as possible. When beginning care, adjustments are relatively frequent to maximize their effect. Healing often takes time, much like if you dropped a brick on your foot, when you take it off, you still need time to heal before it starts feeling better.

Intermediate or Reconstructive Care

Continuing adjustments on a slightly less frequent basis to return the function of your spine to as near as possible to normal. This is the level of care that usually produces the major changes in the function of your spine and nervous system as chronic or underlying subluxations are corrected. This stage will enable you to make more supportive changes regarding every aspect of your lifestyle. Remember: health is a process, not an event!

Advanced or Wellness Care

The lives of most people include ample opportunities to create subluxations. Wellness care involves regular spinal checks and adjustments to continue the improvement in the function of your spine and correct subluxations as you create them. Generally people in this level of care experience greater energy levels, improved ability to concentrate, they become sick less often, they are more able to adapt to stresses and they are overall more healthy and happy; functioning at a higher level.

Types of care

Periodic spinal check-ups are vitally important to maintaining good health, just like eating well and exercising!

How Will I Feel After A Chiropractic Adjustment?

By removing interference to your nervous system, your body is better able to coordinate and heal itself more fully. Most people report a reduction in their symptoms or a warm relaxed feeling after being adjusted. Many people find they have increased energy, a more restful sleep, increased clarity of thought and improved ability to adapt to stress.

Some do not feel any change after an adjustment. This does not mean they are not experiencing the benefits of chiropractic, however, they may not be as consciously aware of the changes in their body as the nerve supply to all the tissues and organs begins to be restored.

A minority of people experience a temporary increase in their discomfort or presenting symptoms. This is usually due to the muscles adapting to the corrections made by the chiropractic adjustments, much like starting a new exercise program.

One of the major functions of your nervous system is to inform you about parts of your body which are not functioning correctly or that need your attention. As you progress through the healing process, you may notice old aches and pains surfacing. This is known as retracing, similar to peeling the layers off of an onion. Retracing may occur as you begin to use your body more fully on your journey through old distortion (compensation) patterns on to a new vibrant state of health!

Chart of Effects of Spinal Misalignments

"The nervous system controls and co-ordinates all organs and structures of the human body" (Gray's Anatomy). Subluxations (misalignments) of spinal vertebrae and discs may cause irritation to the nervous system and may affect the structures, organs, and functions, which may result in the conditions below.

Vertebrae		Structures, Organs, and Functions Affected	Conditions that Follow Pressure on or Interference with these Nerves
Cervical	C1	Blood supply to the head, pituitary gland, scalp, bones of the face, brain, inner & middle ear, sympathetic nervous system	Headaches, nervousness, insomnia, head colds, high blood pressure, migraine, headaches, chronic tiredness, dizziness, vertigo, or any of the problems below
	C2	Eyes, optical nerves, auditory nerves, sinuses, mastoid bones, tongue, forehead	Sinus troubles, allergies, headaches, neck pain
	C3	Cheeks, outer ear, face bones, teeth, diaphragm	Neuralgia, neuritis, headaches, neck pain
	C4	Nose, lips, mouth, eustachian tube	Hay fever, hard of hearing
	C5	Vocal cords, neck glands, & pharynx	Laryngitis, hoarseness, throat conditions, sore throat
	C6	Neck muscles, shoulders, tonsils	Stiff neck, pain in upper arms, tonsillitis
	C7	Thyroid glands, bursae in shoulders, elbows	Bursitis, colds, thyroid conditions
Thoracic	T1	Arms from the elbows down including hands, wrists, & fingers; oesophagus, & trachea	Pain in lower arms, wrists & hands, difficulty swallowing, hiatal hernia, heartburn
	T2	Heart including valves and covering, coronary vessels	Chest pains, tightness or constriction
	T3	Lungs, bronchial tubes, pleura, chest, breast	Asthma, cough, difficulty breathing, congestion, pain between the shoulder blades
	T4	Gall bladder, common duct	Gall bladder conditions, jaundice, shingles
	T5	Liver, solar plexus, blood	Liver conditions, fevers, low blood pressure, poor circulation
	T6	Stomach	Stomach conditions, indigestion
	T7	Pancreas, duodenum	Ulcers, gastritis
	T8	Spleen	Lowered resistance
	T9	Adrenal and supra-renal glands	Allergies, hives, fatigue
	T10	Kidneys	Kidney conditions, hardening of the arteries, chronic tiredness
	T11	Kidneys, ureters	Skin conditions like acne, eczema, boils etc.
	T12	Small intestine, lymph circulation	Gas pains, indigestion, lowered resistance
Lumbar	L1	Large intestines (colon), ileocecal valve, inguinal rings	Constipation, colitis, diarrhoea, ruptures, or hernias
	L2	Appendix, abdomen, upper leg	Appendicitis, cramps, difficult breathing, acidosis, varicose veins
	L3	Sex organs, uterus, bladder, knees	Bladder troubles; menstrual troubles, bed wetting, impotence, many knee pains
	L4	Prostate gland, muscles of lower back, sciatic nerve	Sciatica, painful or frequent (difficult) urination, backaches
	L5	Sciatic nerve, lower legs, ankles, feet	Poor circulation in the legs and feet, weak ankles & arches, weakness in the legs, leg cramps, trouble walking
Sacrum		Hip bones, buttocks	Sacroiliac conditions, pain or soreness in the hips and buttocks, spinal curvature
Coccyx		Rectum, anus	Haemorrhoids (piles), pruritis (itching), pain at end of spine when sitting

The nervous system is complex and only the most significant relationships are shown. Innervation of the spinal nerves in the human body overlap in their supply to different areas and parts of the body as well as differ somewhat in different persons. This chart is a simplification of actual innervation, designed for ease of layman's understanding and general edification and is not meant and should not be construed as anatomically accurate in its specific sense.

Note: The possible symptoms listed on this chart are not meant and should not be construed to mean that all these possible symptoms are produced whenever there is a subluxation at a specific vertebral level or that chiropractic care will correct all of these conditions.

14

An Expectant Parent's Guide to Chiropractic

From the moment of conception, your body goes through a series of remarkable changes.

It is easy for all of us to see postural changes through pregnancy—the centre of gravity changes, the weight of the baby places increased pressure on the spine and pelvis, and towards the end of the pregnancy, changes are seen in the gait pattern—the characteristic "pregnancy waddle." What we cannot see are the millions of different hormonal changes and chemical reactions occurring both in the mother and the developing baby—all of which are controlled and coordinated through the nervous system. Now more than ever, you need a nervous system that responds immediately and accurately to changing requirements in all parts of your body; therefore you need a healthy spine! Chiropractic care prior to conception promotes a more regular menstrual cycle and optimal uterine function. It prepares the body to be strong, supple and as balanced as possible to carry the pregnancy. Restoring proper nerve supply to reproductive organs has helped many couples that thought they were infertile (see *Appendix Three—A Plausible Cause of Infertility Discovered*). And adjusting women through pregnancy is one of the most rewarding parts of our work, because a healthier pregnancy means an easier labour and delivery, and a better transition for the baby into this life!

A person's spine is made of twenty-four moveable bones called vertebrae, plus the sacrum (tailbone), pelvis, and skull. From the brain, nerve impulses travel down the spinal cord and branch out into nerves, exiting between the vertebrae. When the vertebrae become misaligned or unable to move properly, it irritates and interferes with the nerves. The message from the brain is slowed down and the life energy carried by the nerve is unable to reach the organs and tissues at one hundred per cent of its potential (See *Chart of Effects of Spinal Misalignments*). A Doctor of Chiropractic aligns the vertebrae and pelvis through gentle adjustments to the spine, relieving the pressure on the nerves and allowing one hundred per cent of the nerve energy to reach the tissues it serves.

As you gain weight, especially in the abdomen, this exerts a downward, forward pull on the lower spine. This extra weight and changes in your gait can set the stage for backache. Additionally, as labour approaches, your body secretes a hormone called Relaxin, which loosens ligaments. This may exaggerate the effects of an existing spinal or pelvis problem. The positioning of the baby and its movement as well as expansion of the lower part of the ribcage to accommodate your growing baby can also cause discomfort in the ribs and upper portion of the lower back.

According to recent studies, chiropractic care may result in easier pregnancy including increased comfort during the third trimester and delivery, and reduced need for analgesics (pain medication). In one study, women receiving chiropractic care through their first pregnancy had twenty-four per cent shorter labour times and subjects giving birth for the second or third time reported thirty-nine per cent shorter labour times. In another study, the need for analgesics was reduced by fifty per cent in the patients who received adjustments. In addition, eighty-four

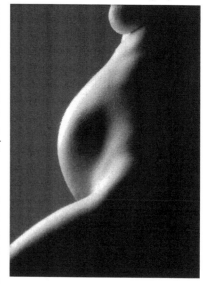

per cent of women report relief of back pain during pregnancy with chiropractic care! And because the sacroiliac joints of the pelvis function better, there is significantly less likelihood of back labour (contractions and sharp pain felt in the lower back during labour) when receiving chiropractic care through pregnancy. Chiropractic care has also been shown to reduce the likelihood of post-partum depression.

As your pregnancy advances, some chiropractic techniques will need to be modified for your comfort. Your Chiropractor is aware of this and will make the necessary changes. In particular, special pregnancy pillows and tables with drop-away pelvic pieces are used to accommodate your growing belly. Side-lying manual (diversified or Gonstead) lumbar or pelvic adjustments should be avoided in the

Copyright Kimberly Mara, Eclipse Photography, 2004

second and third trimester due to patient discomfort and a small risk of disrupting the placental attachment from the uterine wall. A chiropractor trained in the techniques that address uterine constraint or mal-presentations will check for misalignment of the pelvic bones, misalignment of the sacrum and vertebrae, and spasm of the ligaments that support the uterus and help hold the pelvis together.

Body position during delivery is also critical. Any late second stage labour position that denies postural sacral (tailbone) rotation denies the mother and the baby critical pelvic outlet diameter and jams the tip of the sacrum up to four centimetres into the pelvic outlet. In other words, the popular semi-recumbent position that places the labouring woman on her back onto the apex of the sacrum closes off the vital space needed for the baby to get through the pelvic outlet.

This delivery position is the main reason why so many births are traumatic—labour is stalled, the mom becomes fatigued and overwhelmed by pain, so the utilization of epidurals, forceps, episiotomies, vacuum extraction, and caesarean increases. Just consider this analogy: how hard would it be to have a bowel movement while lying on your back? Very hard, and it may not happen at all. This is why squatting is the preferred position—gravity works to help and the pelvic outlet can open to a greater degree. Squatting during delivery results in decreased use of forceps and a shorter second stage of labour than the semi-recumbent position!

Moreover, research has shown that coached pushing in the second stage of labour does not improve the short-term outcome for mothers or babies, except when the baby needs to be born as quickly as possible. Coaching pushing has also been found to potentially increase the amount of pressure on the pelvic floor with subsequent negative consequences such as decreased bladder capacity, less urge to empty the bladder, an overactive bladder muscle, and stress incontinence (leakage of urine). Coaching pushing also involves "breath-holding" (so-called "purple pushing") which can be very tiring, reduces oxygen levels in the mother and baby and increases the risk of tearing. An uncoached or a spontaneous second stage of labour allows the mother to work with the uterine contractions and the foetal expulsion reflex and allows the baby to descend without damage as she gently pushes/breathes the baby out.

We now know that on-going moderate, low-impact weight-bearing exercise during pregnancy can contribute to normal, on-time delivery and improve the likelihood of giving birth to a healthy, heavier baby. Unless there are medical reasons to avoid it, pregnant women can and should exercise moderately for at least thirty minutes on most, if not all, days. Exercise helps women feel better. The calories burned help prevent too much weight gain. Exercise can help pregnant women avoid gestational diabetes; a form of diabetes that sometimes develops during pregnancy. It can help build the stamina needed for labour and delivery. Exercise enhances well being and promotes early recovery after labour and delivery. It's also worth mentioning that exercise can be very helpful in coping with the postpartum period: exercise can help new mothers keep "baby blues" at bay, regain their energy and lose the weight they gained during pregnancy.

Pregnancy Exercise Tips

- Don't exercise for longer than thirty minutes at a time.
- Always include a ten-minute warm-up and a ten-minute cool-down period (in addition to the thirty minutes of exercise).
- Pregnant women should not exercise to exhaustion—being fatigued is okay.
- Avoid forced, passive stretches, such as reaching for your toes or doing hamstring stretches. Pregnancy hormones make your joints looser, so overstretching—which can cause a muscle injury—is a greater risk during pregnancy. Also, avoid sudden jerking or bouncing movements or quick changes in position.
- Limit aerobic activity to the low-impact variety, especially if you weren't exercising regularly before getting pregnant. Brisk walking, swimming, and riding a stationary bicycle are good choices. Keep it moderate (thirty minutes per day), particularly if you weren't exercising before. Ensure weight training is done under proper guidance.
- Measure your heart rate at peak activity to be sure you are not exceeding 140 beats per minute.
- Avoid overheating: drink plenty of water, and don't exercise in hot, humid conditions.
- Avoid activities that put you at high risk for injury, such as horseback riding or downhill skiing.
- Avoid sports in which you could get hit in the abdomen.
- Especially after the third month, avoid exercises that require you to lie flat on your back for an extended period of time since this can reduce your heart rate, lower your blood pressure, cause dizziness, and may reduce blood flow to baby.
- Never scuba dive because it can cause dangerous gas bubbles in the baby's circulatory system.
- Before starting any new exercise routine, always check with your health care provider.
- Stop exercising immediately and consult your midwife or doctor if any of the following symptoms occur during or after exercise:

  - Bleeding
  - Cramping
  - Faintness and/or dizziness
  - Elevated blood pressure
  - Severe joint pain.

Here's an easy exercise to get you started—to strengthen stomach and back muscles and reduce stress from the growing baby (see also *Returning the Uterus, Perineum and Abdominal Muscles to Normal More Quickly*).

Starting Position:

1) Lie flat on your back with your knees bent (this can also be done standing if you are uncomfortable on your back).
2) If needed, place a small pillow under your neck and/or lower back for support. Make sure you maintain a small curve in your neck to reduce the likelihood of strain.

Pelvic Tilt:

1) Assume starting position. You may want to make sure you haven't eaten for an hour or so before doing this exercise for comfort.
2) Pull in abdominal and buttock muscles (this should flatten the lower back). Imagine you are peeling your buttocks and spine up off the floor, slowly, vertebra-by-vertebra, to approximately bra-strap level (as long as there is no pain or tension felt in your neck).
3) Hold, breathe out, and count to five.
4) Relax. Inhale. Roll down slowly, and with control, vertebra-by-vertebra.
5) Repeat five times.

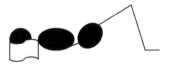

Additional Hints to Help Prevent Pregnancy Backache

- Stand erect—do not allow your belly to sag.
- Change positions often to ease lower back strain.
- When lifting, bend your knees and keep your back straight.
- Consult your Chiropractor for exercises to reduce lower back strain (an easy one to start with is the pelvic tilt shown overleaf).
- Your mattress should be supportive and comfortable.
- Sleep on your side with a pillow between your knees.
- Adequate rest is essential.

- Keep daily chores manageable. Seek those who can most help you make this experience meaningful. Whether it's a friend to walk with to the pool, a doula to help with your labour plan, your mother offering to watch the kids or help clean the kitchen, take advantage of the help around you.
- Know your limits—whether you're working throughout your pregnancy and/or have other children to care for, try not to overdo it.
- Practice good postural habits.
- Plan and do regular exercise.
- Kegel exercises are a great way to prepare and tone the pelvic floor muscles for delivery, and can be done anytime. To do Kegels, contract the muscles around your urethra and vagina—imagine you're trying to prevent yourself from urinating. Hold for several seconds, then release. Repeat sets of ten, several times each day.
- Have regular spinal check-ups; they are an important part of preventative health care.

Other Factors to Consider in Maintaining a Healthy Pregnancy

- Proper nutrition is essential including adequate intake of folic acid, good sources of protein and iron, calcium-rich foods, and lots of fruits and vegetables.
- Drink plenty of pure water to keep well hydrated.
- Avoid eating too much sugar and sweets including fruit drinks as they can cause you (and the baby) to gain excessive weight.
- Research has found that a pregnant woman can help protect the health of her child by avoiding:

    - Smoking and second-hand smoke
    - Alcohol
    - Excessive caffeine (e.g. tea, coffee and cola)
    - Unnecessary exposure to x-rays (especially in the first trimester)
    - Unnecessary medication (including over-the-counter remedies)
    - Foods with chemical additives, artificial sweeteners, and artificial ingredients.
    - See *Things You Should Do and Should Not Do During Pregnancy*.

Regular exercise, good nutrition, and periodic spinal adjustments can make pregnancy the pleasant, exciting experience you want it to be! Pregnancy should be an opportunity to reflect on your family's plans and dreams—not a time to struggle with pain. Preparing for a new baby is a daunting challenge for even the most organized mothers-to-be. So, during this meaningful time, be proactive: work to prevent backache before it affects your peace of mind or distracts you from focusing on your family's well being. Chiropractic care is safe and natural, simply removing interference to your body's own controlling and healing ability.

[Adapted from an article by Martha Collins, DC
http://www.planetchiropractic.com]

15

Chiropractic and Pregnancy: Greater Comfort and Safer Births

Chapter by Jeanne Ohm, DC

Chiropractic care in pregnancy is an essential ingredient to your pre-natal care choices.

How Can Chiropractic Add Comfort?

A large percent of all pregnant women experience back discomfort/ pain during pregnancy. This is due to the rapid growth of the baby and interference to your body's normal structural adaptations to that growth. Pre-existing, unnoticed imbalances in your spine and pelvis become overtaxed during these times. The added stresses lead to discomfort and difficulty while performing routine, daily activities. Chiropractic care throughout pregnancy can relieve and even prevent the common discomforts experienced in pregnancy. Specific adjustments eliminate these stresses in your spine, restore balance to your pelvis and result in greater comfort and lifestyle improvements.

Comfort For Your Baby, Too.

As your baby develops, your uterus enlarges to accommodate the rapid growth. So long as the pelvis is in a balanced state, the ligaments connected to the uterus maintain an equalized, supportive suspension for the uterus. If your pelvis is out of balance in any way, these ligaments become torqued and twisted, causing a condition known as constraint to your uterus. This constraint limits the space of the developing baby. Any compromised position for the baby throughout pregnancy will affect his or her optimal development. Conditions such as torticollis occur because a baby's space was cramped in utero.

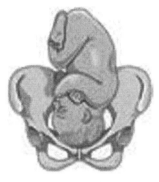 If the woman's uterus is constrained as birth approaches, the baby is prevented from getting into the best possible position for birth. Even if the baby is in the desirable head down position, often times, constraint to the uterus affects the baby's head from moving into the ideal presentation for delivery. The head may be slightly tilted off to one side or even more traumatically, present in the posterior position. Any baby position even slightly off during birth will slow down labour, and add pain to both the mother and baby. Many women have been told that their babies were too big, or labour "just slowed down" when it was really the baby's presentation interfering with the normal process and progression. Avoidable interventions are implemented turning a natural process into an operative one. Doctors of Chiropractic work specifically with your pelvis throughout pregnancy restoring a state of balance and creating an environment for an easier, safer delivery.

Preparing For A Safer Birth

Dystocia is defined as difficult labour and is something every woman wants to avoid. In addition to the pain and exhaustion caused by long, difficult labours, dystocia leads to multiple, medical interventions, which may be physically and emotionally traumatic to both you and your baby. Some of these interventions are the administering of Pitocin [synthetic oxytocin], the use of epidurals, painful episiotomies, forceful pulling on the baby's fragile spine, vacuum extraction, forceps and perhaps even caesarean sections. Each of these procedures carries a high risk of injury to you, your baby, or both! However, all of these procedures used to hasten the delivery process can be avoided if delivery goes more smoothly to begin with.

When reviewing the obstetric texts, pelvic imbalance and its resulting effects on your uterus and your baby's position cause the reported reasons for dystocia. Chiropractic care throughout pregnancy restores balance to your pelvic muscles and ligaments and therefore leads to safer and easier deliveries for you and your baby. Additionally, the chiropractic adjustment removes interference to the nervous system allowing your uterus to function at its maximum potential. Published studies have indicated that chiropractic care does in fact reduce labour time.

[Chiropractors] offer specific analysis and adjustments for your special needs in pregnancy. You and your baby's continued safety and comfort is primary in our care. This pregnancy, offer yourself the best! Include the many benefits chiropractic offers in your pre-natal care choices. Call for your individual consultation. Give you and your baby the opportunity for a more comfortable pregnancy and a safer, easier birth!

The I.C.P.A. is the oldest and largest organization of its kind. Its purpose is to offer research, training and education because all children need chiropractic care. For additional information visit the I.C.P.A. at www.icpa4kids.com or call 610 565-2360

16

How to Care for Your Spine— Good Pregnancy Body Mechanics

Good posture during pregnancy involves training your body to stand, walk, sit and lie in positions where the least strain is placed on your back.

Daily activities can put stress on your back and neck, causing pain. Although your growing belly may make you feel like you are going to topple, there are several steps you can take to maintain good posture and proper body mechanics during pregnancy. Included here are some tips so that changing how you perform simple everyday activities (the position in which you hold your body while standing, sitting or lying down), you can lessen the stress, avoiding injury and pain.

Standing

Hold your head up straight with your chin in. Do not tilt your head forward, backward or sideways. Make sure your ear lobes are in line with the middle of your shoulders. Keep your shoulder blades back and your chest forward. Point your feet in the same direction, with your weight balanced evenly on both feet. The arches of your feet should be supported with low-heeled (but not flat) shoes to prevent stress on your back. You can also try standing with one-foot forward and knees slightly bent (not locked straight) and be sure to alternate feet.

Avoid standing in the same position for a long time. If you need to stand for long periods in front of a table, adjust the height of the table to a comfortable level if possible. Try to elevate one foot by resting it on a stool or box (the cupboard under your sink also works well). A diagonal stance works well at home while washing dishes, brushing your teeth, etc. Change foot position every five to fifteen minutes.

Sitting

Get knees level or slightly higher than the hips with back support (such as a small, rolled-up towel or a lumbar roll) at the curve of your back. Keep your hips and knees at a right angle (use a foot rest or stool if necessary). Your legs should not be crossed and your feet should be flat on the floor.

Sit up with your back straight and your shoulders back. Your buttocks should touch the back of your chair. Try to avoid sitting in the same position for more than thirty minutes. At work, adjust your chair height and workstation so you can sit up close to your work. Rest your elbows and arms on your chair or desk, keeping your shoulders relaxed. When sitting in a chair that rolls and pivots, don't twist at the waist while sitting. Instead, turn your whole body.

When standing up from the sitting position, move to the front of the seat of your chair. Stand up by straightening your legs. Avoid bending forward at your waist.

Driving

Use a back support such as a lumbar roll in the curve of your back. Your knees should be at the same level or higher than your hips. Move the seat close to the steering wheel, but not too close. In general, your seat should be close enough to allow your knees to bend and your feet to reach the pedals. Your belly should be at least ten inches from the steering wheel, if possible (this will depend upon your height). You may need to move the seat back to get in and out of the vehicle comfortably. The last month of pregnancy, when your belly is likely to be closer than ever to the steering wheel, ride in the passenger's seat when possible.

Always wear both the lap and shoulder safety belts. Place the lap belt under your abdomen, as low on your hips as possible and across your upper thighs. Never place the belt above your abdomen. Place the shoulder belt between your breasts. Adjust the shoulder and lap belts as snug as possible. Also, always make sure the headrest is in the ideal position to prevent whiplash.

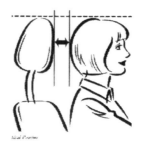

If your vehicle is equipped with an air bag, it is very important to wear your shoulder and lap belts. In addition, always sit back at least ten inches away from the site where the air bag is stored. On the driver's side, the air bag is located in the steering wheel. When driving, pregnant women should adjust the steering wheel so that it is tilted toward the chest and away from the head and abdomen.

Reaching

Use a diagonal stance to get items from above. Get your body as close as possible to the object you need.

Stand on a stool to reach above shoulder level. Make sure you have a good idea of how heavy the object is you are going to lift. Use two hands to lift.

Bending

You can bend this way to get light objects out.

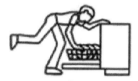

Or get down on one knee to get to low levels.

Pushing

Pushing is easier on your back than pulling. Use your arms and legs to start the push.

Pulling

Keep the handle next to your side. Do not twist your lower back while pulling.

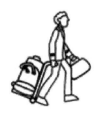

Carrying

Two small objects may be easier to handle than one large one.

Keep the load close at all times.

Lifting

Before you lift an object, make sure you have firm footing. Lifting with your heels off the floor can cause you to lose your balance.

A diagonal stance will provide you with the stability you need for lifting. Stand with a wide stance close to the object you are trying to pick up and keep your feet firm on the ground. Tighten your stomach muscles and lift the object using your leg muscles.

Lift with your legs, not your back! Straighten your knees in a steady motion. Don't jerk the object up to your body. Stand completely upright without twisting. Always move your feet forward when lifting an object. Avoid lifting heavy objects above waist level. A hand on your leg will help support your upper body. Use the diagonal stance to balance the load.

A knee on the bumper will give you the leverage you need to safely get objects out of the trunk.

To lower the object, place your feet as you did to lift. Tighten your stomach muscles and bend your hips and knees.

Pivoting

Move your shoulders, hips, and feet at the same time. Keep the load in front of you.

Sleeping

Sleeping flat on your back produces fifty-five pounds of disc pressure on your spine. Sleeping flat on your back puts the full weight of your uterus on your back, intestines, and your inferior vena cava (the vein that transports blood from your lower body back to your heart). Back sleeping can also increase your risk for backaches and haemorrhoids, inefficient digestion, and impaired breathing and circulation. Lying on your back in the second and third trimester can also cause changes in blood pressure. For some women, it can cause a drop in blood pressure that can make them feel very dizzy; for others, it can cause an unwanted increase in blood pressure. Because your liver is on the right side of your body, lying on the left side also helps keep the uterus off that large organ.

No matter what position you lie in, a pillow should be under your head, but not your shoulders, and should be a thickness that allows your head to be in a normal 'neutral' position to avoid straining your back. You may also want to put a pillow between your legs for support. There are several special "pregnancy" pillows on the market that may help you sleep better. Sleeping on your left side with a pillow between your knees and/or a body pillow reduces the disc pressure to forty pounds. It also optimizes blood flow back to the heart, as the inferior vena cava is located slightly more on the right side of the spine.

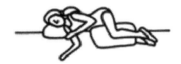

Select a firm mattress and box spring set that does not sag. If necessary, place a board under your mattress. You can also place the mattress on the floor temporarily if necessary. If you have always slept on a soft surface, it may be more painful to change to a hard surface. Try to do what is most comfortable for you. Try using a back support (lumbar support, rolled sheet or towel) at night to make you more comfortable and to maintain the natural curve in your back.

When standing up from the lying position, turn on your side, draw up both knees and swing your legs on/over the side of the bed. Sit up by pushing yourself up with your hands. Avoid bending forward at your waist.

Relaxing

This position works well while watching TV.

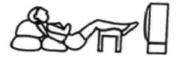

17

Pre-natal Yoga

Chapter by Janice Clarfield

The word yoga is translated from Sanskrit to mean union, that is union of the body, mind and spirit.

What is Pre-natal Yoga?

From a yogic point of view, life is to be enjoyed and experienced fully. With pregnancy, there is more joy. Pre-natal yoga is the nurturing activity undertaken when time is spent (a little or a lot) to gently relax, release and attune to your body and your rapidly growing baby within. The natural, vital and restorative energies of the body and mind are enhanced through gentle yoga postures.

When pregnant, one feels the strains of the ever-changing body, particularly the new demands upon the back. Yoga work counterbalances the growing abdomen, promotes and helps maintain good posture. Stretching while strengthening helps to release the pelvic opening in preparation for birth. Toning the pelvic floor allows for a more controlled birthing, lessens complications and enhances postnatal healing.

Breath work is practiced in preparation for responding to labour by coordinating with the rhythms of contractions. Breathing awareness is essential for relaxation, comfort and confidence.

Just being in your body that is home for two is yoga. Your pregnant body is naturally and miraculously in a state of enhanced energy and creativity. Taking time to pause from the stream of day-to-day activity to connect with your body enables you to experience and enjoy these augmented senses.

With hormonal changes, emotions are also heightened. Whether they are in the realm of joy or sorrow, love or anger, feelings may be experienced with surprising depth and in rapidly changing rhythms. Noticing and allowing yourself to feel your emotions fully has a positive effect on your health and therefore on your baby's health too.

All women experience some fear of labour. A simple foundation in yoga prepares you to face childbirth with courage. To be relaxed and confident during labour reduces fear, tension and fatigue. Flexibility and calm ease the birthing process, thus reducing pain and increasing the joy of giving birth.

While practicing yoga, your relationship with your baby deepens—physically, mentally and spiritually. It is a time to be mindful that you are engaged in the creation of new life, and to be attentive to the impact of this major life passage. Taking time in this way allows the quickly passing nine months to be cherished.

Even if you have never practiced yoga before, being pregnant can provide the motivation for beginning this healthful practice which will hasten your recovery, and you can carry on long after your baby is born. You will find that your practice will become a source of strength and love, during and after pregnancy.

18

New Baby Ergonomics—
Tips To Prevent The Aches And Pains
That Can Come with Becoming a New
Parent

Mother Nature sure has an odd sense of humour. Why else could it be that at exactly the time a women most needs to be strong and resilient—when she's caring for a brand-new baby—she is most vulnerable to strains and injury?

When a woman comes home from hospital, she's still in a physical state that's similar to when she was pregnant. After the birth, you're carrying some additional weight, your breasts are enlarged and your belly muscles are weak. On top of that, you still have the hormone Relaxin in your system, loosening up your joints and connective tissue.

All of those might clear up on their own were it not for the fact that your mothering instincts will lead you to putting baby's comfort ahead of your own. This often means that you're slouching at feedings or twisting awkwardly to lift baby from her bassinet or car seat. Some moms are afraid of moving a muscle when the baby's asleep in their arms, even if their shoulders are cramping up and elbows have fallen asleep, for fear of waking their little one. These ergonomically incorrect moves may seem to be for baby's benefit, but if you wind up in pain—or worse, out of commission—that's not good for either of you!

Here's a guide to safer posture and movements you can use every day with your baby:

Snuggle Front and Centre

Carrying your little one seems like it should be the most natural thing in the world. But remember how that extra weight at the front of your body gave you a sore back when you were pregnant? The same thing can happen when you've got a baby in your arms. To minimize strain, it is important that women improve their posture and look at how they're standing and holding themselves.

Imagine a fishing line pulling you up from your sternal notch (the bump on the upper part of your breastbone). This will make your chest come up and your shoulders come down with your chin tucked in. Now it's time to work on how best to hold your baby. Carrying her close to your body is safest; avoid holding her with outstretched arms for longer than it takes to say, "Whee!"

Walking around with baby's car seat can be awkward, to say the least, so keep those occasions to a minimum. If you have to carry it, carry it in front as opposed to off to the side. Stroller travel systems, or snap-and-go stroller frames, which allow you to transfer baby quickly from your vehicle to her own set of wheels, are a big help in easing that burden.

When you need to free up your arms, front carriers or slings come in handy. As with everything else, just be sure not to overdo. The risk of a front carrier is putting the baby in it and then trying to do everything around your house. That will cause strain. Additionally, there is evidence to suggest that babies who spend a lot of time in an upright position before they have adequate muscle strength and coordination are more at risk of a spinal condition called spondylolisthesis due to the compressive forces on their lower spine. Remember: the dusting and the dishes can wait until later—so ease up on yourself, and enjoy your time with your little one.

Diapering Don'ts

Your change table, or any other surface you use for diaper duty, should be at waist height, allowing you to keep your back straight and strong. A too-low table can be remedied by placing wooden blocks underneath. Similarly, if bath time leaves you with an aching back, placing baby's tub on a broad, sturdy countertop or table will allow you to stand up straight the entire time.

Note: Avoid sharply bringing baby's legs up and excessively flexing her mid-back as this may also cause the baby repetitive strain in her hips, legs, and spine. It is best to try to lift her only a little bit and then wiggle the fresh diaper underneath her, or use your free hand underneath to lift her buttocks (rather than pull up by baby's ankles or legs) then slide the clean diaper underneath.

Stroller Safety

Strollers are great for giving your back a break—when you use them properly. As you walk behind the stroller, your elbows should be slightly bent, back straight. Ideally, your stroller should have adjustable handles so that you, your spouse and other caregivers can easily raise or lower the handles to waist level—the optimal position for ergonomic ease. In case you've inherited a stroller with fixed handles that are too low for your comfort, check your favourite baby supply store for handle extenders.

Now that you've nailed the stroller walk, don't blow it by bending over to transfer baby in and out. Instead of hunching your back, kneel on one knee to get down to baby's level, and then straighten your legs to stand up.

Blissful Mealtimes

Whether you're feeding with the breast or bottle, mealtimes are wonderful for bonding with baby. But getting feedings to feel right takes practice, and those first weeks home, especially, can be filled with questions: "Is my baby latched on well? Getting enough milk?" While relaxation may be the last thing on your mind, it's important for you to know how to make yourself comfortable.

To help baby latch on correctly, lactation consultants emphasize the importance of bringing baby up to your breast, instead of the other way around. That advice is ergonomically sound, as well. In this regard, nursing pillows are great, to bring the baby up to breast level. Sometimes it may be necessary to put another pillow underneath the nursing pillow. It depends on your height.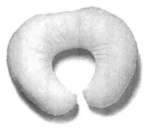

Placing a small pillow between baby's head and the crook of your arm can also help avoid discomfort. The inside of your arm is highly clustered with nerves and, hence, extremely sensitive. The good news is, a little padding is all most women need to relieve the pressure. Because everyone is built differently, you'll have to experiment a bit to find your optimal nursing set-up. Some women find that sitting in a chair or sofa with an armrest is best; for others, crossing one leg over the other is the perfect way to give baby a boost. Consciously keep your shoulders down and relaxed. And use a small pillow behind your lower back to support the natural curve there if needed. Not sure of your set-up? Ask your partner or a friend to take a picture. Seeing what you look like can help you pinpoint problem areas.

For breastfeeding moms, a breast that feels full or becomes leaky usually acts as a built-in reminder to switch sides when you're feeding the baby—a good habit that staves off strain and repetitive stress injuries. A safety pin on your nursing bra that you switch from side to side after feedings also works well. However, if you're bottle-feeding, you might need additional help to remember. Try using a soft, loose bracelet or ponytail elastic that you can switch from one wrist to another. Switching sides when feeding baby is also good for baby's neurological development, stimulating both sides of his body, and providing closeness for bonding with skin-to-skin contact.

Lower Before You Lift

The saying, "lift with your legs," isn't just a cliché; it's a great back-saving tip. Prepare to lift baby by planting your feet wide apart to create a sturdy base of support. Keep your spine in a neutral position—you'll know you're doing it right if it feels almost like you have a stiff back. Then, bend your knees to lower yourself to baby's level, and straighten them to lift. If you need to bend down and to one side, shift sideways by moving your feet, not by twisting your back.

If you begin to experience back pain, chiropractic treatment may help. Chiropractic is a safe and effective way to relieve pain in the joints, muscles and nerves along the spinal column.

[Adapted from "New Baby Ergonomics: Tricks to Prevent the Aches and Strains that Come with the Territory," article by SE Martin in *Today's Parent Baby and Toddler*]

19

Babies and Chiropractic: A Parent's Guide

A healthy spine and nervous system, working at its
very best can help anyone at anytime in their life!

How Could My Baby Have Spinal Problems?

Even today's 'natural' childbirth methods can affect a child's spine! The birth
process and eager hands pulling and twisting can put a great deal of pressure on
the spinal nerves and muscles of the infant's neck (up to eighty pounds in some
studies). In a difficult delivery, damage to the delicate tissues of the spine may
occur, especially when vacuum extraction or forceps are used. While forceps
injuries may be less common today, vacuum extraction can do just as much
damage—120 pounds of pressure goes through the baby's head and neck to
literally suck the baby out of the mother (decapitation can occur at 140 pounds
of pressure, to give you an idea of the high forces involved). In addition, a severe
drop in temperature, loud noises, often accompanies a newborn's introduction to
the world and other 'stressful' stimuli including the administration of drugs and
anaesthesia can have a profound effect on the nervous system of a newborn.

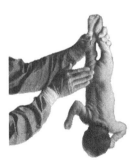

Changing diapers may also place undue stress on the baby's mid-back (thoracic spine). Raising the infant's legs with one hand to place the diaper underneath can cause repetitive stress to these spinal joints. Spinal problems can also occur as a result of the frequent falls suffered by young infants in the first months of life. A fall from a bed, a sudden stop in an automobile, or any significant unsupported movement of the head and neck in an infant can induce excessive movement in the spine causing subluxations. At the other end of the spine, the act of learning to walk, and the number of simple falls encountered in this way, can induce trauma to the lower spinal segments and to the large sacroiliac joints of the pelvis.

What Causes a Subluxation?

Small traumas such as spills, falls, and accidents (especially when learning to crawl and walk) can create misalignments in the child's forming spine and pelvis leading to: poor posture, in-coordination, poor concentration, scoliosis (curvature of the spine), as well as symptoms such as headaches, neck pain, shoulder pain, growing pains, back and leg pains. These spinal misalignments may have a cumulative effect leading to chronic problems in adulthood.

The nervous system is so important that the first cells to differentiate at about seven hours after conception become the brain and spinal cord! The spinal bones called vertebrae protect the nervous system, which controls every function of the body. When a vertebra is misaligned, it can irritate or put pressure on the spinal nerves. This is called a subluxation. The communication between your nervous system (your brain, spinal cord and spinal nerves) and your body becomes hampered and may cause countless problems.

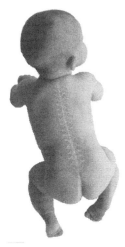

The spine of a child is somewhat different from the fully developed spine of an adult. The vertebrae of a child's spine have abundant cartilage, which eventually converts to bone (ossifies) as the spine continues to develop. Ossification of these cartilaginous sections continues at least until the middle of the second decade of life. The strength of a child's spinal vertebrae is derived, to a significant degree, from the elasticity of this cartilaginous tissue. Because the spine is fragile and developing, it needs to be attended to in order to fix a problem before a child reaches maturity.

The young spine also has a high degree of ligament laxity, which permits a greater degree of motion of individual vertebral structures. It is this ligament laxity that makes adjustment of a child's spine possible with very little pressure and therefore without placing the structures under any significant stress that might be likely to cause harm.

Is it Safe to Adjust My Baby's Spine?

First, your Doctor of Chiropractic will perform a thorough examination of your child to determine if he/she has spinal or pelvis subluxation(s). If subluxations are found, gentle, specific Chiropractic adjustments will be performed to correct them. Baby spinal adjusting techniques are different from those used on adults or older children—they are designed to further protect the developing spinal structures. Because of the flexibility of the developing spine and the size of a child's spinal joints, any adjustive thrust is kept to a minimum. Adjustments to newborns and children contain only ounces of force. However, that force is carefully directed into the spine to facilitate health and remove subluxations. We adjust babies as soon after birth as possible, to alleviate subluxations caused by in utero constraint and the difficult journey down through the birth canal.

How Do I Know if My Baby Needs Chiropractic?

Unless a child has an obvious problem, it can be difficult for parents to recognize when a child has spinal subluxations. There are some signs, however, which parents may look for which can be an indicator of an infant with a spinal problem including: the child's head consistently being tilted to one side; restricted head or neck motion to one side; disturbed sleeping patterns where the child sleeps for only an hour or two at a time; feeding difficulties in the young infant, for example, the infant may have difficulty nursing at the breast on one particular side; and the presence of any of the symptoms of ill-health mentioned previously. Nerve interference from subluxations is implicated in many common childhood health problems such as: sucking dysfunction, colic, irritability, unexplained crying, recurrent ear infections, frequent colds, headaches, asthma, lack of appetite, poor digestion, constipation, stomach aches, so called 'growing pains', back aches, bed-wetting, poor general health, and fatigue.

As you make decisions about your baby's health care and are confronted with the issues of antibiotics, vaccinations, and the growing use of behaviour-altering drugs, consult with your Doctor of Chiropractic. Seek accurate information and make an informed choice. First make sure your child has the best chance to be all that he/she can be by having a system free from subluxations and nerve interference.

Family care can start from the very beginning of a lifetime. Babies can benefit when their mothers receive chiropractic care during pregnancy. And children benefit when they receive safe, gentle, natural chiropractic care—there is no better way to get a head start in life! As you know, chiropractic care is not a cure for anything—it is a system of wellness to help us be who we're supposed to be.

References and Resources

1. "Give Your Baby a Better Start—With Exercise." Short Article. *American Journal of Obstetrics and Gynaecology.* (2000) Vol 183 (6): 1484-1488.
2. Almeida ECS, Nogueira AA et al. "Caesarean Section as a Cause of Chronic Pelvic Pain." *International Journal of Gynaecology.* (2002) Vol 79: 101-104.
3. Bagnell KG. (2005). *Pre-Natal Chiropractic Care.* Instant Publisher.com: USA.
4. Bagnell KG. "How to Explain Chiropractic Care to the Mother To Be." Handout.
5. Bagnell KG. and Bagnell L (2006). *Relieving Common Complaints of Pregnancy, Naturally.* E-Book.
6. Balaskas J. (1992). *Active Birth.* Harvard Common Press: Boston, MA.
7. Balon J et al. "A Comparison of Active and Simulated Chiropractic Manipulation as Adjunctive Treatment for Childhood Asthma." *The New England Journal of Medicine.* (1998, October) Vol 339: 15.
8. Baumgarder DJ, Muehl P et al. "Effect of Labour Epidural Anaesthesia on Breast-Feeding of Healthy Full-Term Newborns Delivered Vaginally." *Journal of the American Board of Family Practice.* (2003, January) Vol 16: 7-13.
9. Belair O. Pregnancy and Herbs Handout.
10. Berg G, Hammer M et al. "Lower Back Pain During Pregnancy." *Obstetrics and Gynecology.* (1988) 71: 701-775.
11. Berman M. (2005, July 27th). "Homeopathy for Pregnancy, Birth, and Post-Partum." Lecture presented, Sechelt, BC.
12. Bromberger P, Lawrence J et al. "The Influence of Intrapartum Antibiotics on the Clinical Spectrum of Early-Onset Group B Streptococcal Infection in Term Infants." *Paediatrics,* (2000, August) Vol 106: 244-250.
13. Buckley SJ. "Ecstatic Birth: The Hormonal Blueprint of Labour." *Mothering Magazine.* (2002: March-April) 51-59.
14. Clapp F, Kim H et al. "Continuing Regular Exercise During Pregnancy: Effect of Exercise Volume on Foetoplacental Growth." *American Journal of Obstetrics and Gynaecology.* (2002) Vol 186: 142-147.

15. Clarfield J. "Prenatal Yoga." *www.urbanyoga.ca.*

16. Collins M. "Pregnancy and Chiropractic." *www.planetchiropractic.com.*

17. Cook M. "Pregnancy Massage." www.ccx.net/massage.

18. Costei AM, Kozer E et al. "Perinatal Outcome Following Third Trimester Exposure to Paroxetine." *Archives of Paediatric and Adolescent Medicine.* (2002, November) Vol 156 (11): 1129-1132.

19. Davies NJ. (1997). *Chiropractic and Osteopathic Paediatrics Reader.* RMIT University: Dept. of Chiropractic, Osteopathy and Complementary Medicine.

20. de Inocenio J. "Musculoskeletal Pain in Primary Paediatric Care: Analysis of 1000 Consecutive General Paediatric Clinic Visits." *Paediatrics.* (1998, December) Vol. 102 No. 6.

21. Diakow P, Gladsby T et al. "Back Pain During Pregnancy and Labour." *Journal of Manipulative and Physiological Therapeutics.* (1991) Vol 14: 116-118.

22. Dick-Read G. (2004). *Childbirth Without Fear.* Pinter and Martin Ltd.: London.

23. Dik N, Tate R et al. "Risk of Physician-Diagnosed Asthma in the First 6 Years of Life." *Journal of Asthma* (2000) Vol 37: 589-594.

24. DiLeo J. "Sleeping Positions During Pregnancy." *www.babyzone.com.*

25. Douglas A. (2000). *The Mother of All Pregnancy Books: An All Canadian Guide to Conception, Birth, and Everything in Between.* MacMillan Canada: Etobicoke, ON

26. Ehrenberg HM, Dierker L et al. "Prevalence of Maternal Obesity in an Urban Center." *American Journal of Obstetrics and Gynaecology.* (2002, November) Vol 187(5): 1189-1192.

27. Eisenberg A, Murkoff HE et al. (2002). 3rd ed. *What to Expect When You're Expecting.* Workman Publishing Company, Inc: USA.

28. Eldor J. "Women Advised to Stay Mobile During Childbirth." The National Childbirth Trust. *Reuters Health.* (2002, September 24).

29. England P and Horowitz R. (1998). *Birthing from Within.* Partera Press: Albuquerque.

30. Fallon J. "The Effect of Chiropractic Treatment on Pregnancy and Labour: A Comprehensive Study." *Proceedings of the World Federation of Chiropractic.* (1991) 24-31.

31. Foti T, Davids J et al. "A Biomechanical Analysis of Gait During Pregnancy." *The Journal of Bone and Joint Surgery.* (2000) Vol 82: 625-632.

32. French R. "Please Hands Off!!! The Importance of Having a Non-Invasive Birth Process." *International Chiropractic Paediatric Association Newsletter.* (2002, January-February).

33. Gaskin IM. (2003). *Ina May's Guide to Childbirth.* Bantam.

34. Gottlieb B. ed. (1995). *New Choices in Natural Healing*. Rodale Press, Inc: Emmaus, PA.

35. Gottlieb M. "Neglected Spinal Cord, Brain Stem and Musculoskeletal Injuries Stemming from Birth Trauma." *Journal of Manipulative and Physiological Therapeutics*. (1993) Vol 16(8).

36. Gray H. (2000). *Anatomy of the Human Body*. Philadelphia: Lea & Febiger, 1918.

37. Grunnet-Nilsson N and Wiberg J. "Infantile Colic And Chiropractic Spinal Manipulation." *Archive Of Disease In Childhood*. (2001 September) 85(3): 268-268.

38. Hatch M, Levin B et al. "Maternal Leisure-Time Exercise and Timely Delivery." *American Journal of Public Health*. (1998) Vol 88: 1528-1533.

39. Helland I, Smith L et al. "Maternal Supplementation With Very-Long-Chain n-3 Fatty Acids During Pregnancy and Lactation Augments Children's IQ at Four Years of Age." *Paediatrics*, (2003, January): Vol. 111 No. 1 e39-e44.

40. Honein MA, Paulozzi LJ et al. "Family History, Maternal Smoking and Clubfoot: An Indication of a Gene-Environment Interaction." *American Journal of Epidemiology*. (2000) Vol 152(7): 658-665.

41. http://bmj.bmjjournals.com/cgi/content/abstract/327/7411/368

42. http://eatmoreherbs.com/

43. http://en.wikipedia.org/wiki/Folic_acid

44. http://office.microsoft.com/clipart/

45. http://parenting.ivillage.com/pregnancy/plabor/0,,80mq,00.html

46. http://parenting.ivillage.com/pregnancy/topics/0,,4rpv,00.html

47. http://www.abchomeopathy.com/

48. http://www.allnatural.net/herbpages/dandelion.shtml

49. http://www.alternative-healthzine.com/html/

50. http://www.asklenore.info/breastfeeding/herbs.html

51. http://www.babycenter.com

52. http://www.babyfit.com/

53. http://www.babyguide.ca

54. http://www.bcchiro.com/

55. http://www.bellymasking.com/

56. http://www.bfar.org/bthistle.shtml

57. http://www.birthplan.com

58. http://www.birthwaves.com

59. http://www.botanical.com/botanical/mgmh/f/fennel01.html

60. http://www.bradleybirth.com/

61. http://www.breastfeeding.com/all_about/all_about_fenugreek.html

62. http://www.breastfeedingonline.com

63. http://www.bygpub.com/natural/natural-childbirth.htm
64. http://www.bygpub.com/natural/pregnancy.htm
65. http://www.ccx.net/massage
66. http://www.chiropediatrics.com/
67. http://www.chiropracticgateway.com/gateway-users/index.aspx
68. http://www.chiroweb.com/find/tellmeabout/women.html
69. http://www.drbarbarasturm.com/
70. http://www.drugdigest.org/DD/PrintablePages/herbMonograph/0,11475, 552733,00.html
71. http://www.eclipsephotography.ca/
72. http://www.econetwork.net/~wildmansteve/Plants.Folder/
73. http://www.expectantmothersguide.com/library/houston/bonding.htm
74. http://www.gardenguides.com/
75. http://www.having-a-baby.com/mopb_us.htm
76. http://www.healthy.net/scr/article.asp?ID=1869
77. http://www.herbalremedies.com/14155.html
78. http://www.hypnobabies.com/
79. http://www.HypnoBirthing.com
80. http://www.iblce.org/
81. http://www.icpa4kids.com/
82. http://www.icpa4kids.org/research/chiropractic/breastfeeding.htm
83. http://www.inamay.com/
84. http://www.innvista.com/health/herbs/comfrey.htm
85. http://www.mamashealth.com
86. http://www.mercola.com
87. http://www.ott.igs.net/~laleche/
88. http://www.pampers.com/en_CA/content/type/101/contentId/5691.do
89. http://www.patientmedia.com
90. http://www.planetc1.com/
91. http://www.pregnancy.org/
92. http://www.pregnancyweekly.com
93. http://www.prenatalparenting.com/philosophy/fetal.html
94. http://www.primary.net/~gic/herb/alfalfa.htm
95. http://www.purplesage.org.uk/profiles/blackhaw.htm
96. http://www.rosenet.org/familychiro/posture.htm
97. http://www.susunweed.com/Article_Pregnancy_Problems.htm
98. http://www.todaysparent.com/lifeasparent/yourhealth/
99. http://www.todaysparent.com/pregnancybirth/
100. http://www.truestarhealth.com/Notes/2135002.html
101. http://www.unassistedchildbirth.com/faith.htm
102. http://www.urbanyoga.ca
103. http://www.viable-herbal.com/singles/herbs/s445.htm

104. http://www.vitacost.com/science/hn/Herb/Red_Raspberry.htm
105. http://www.webmd.com/content/article/51/40819.htm
106. http://www.westcoastfamilies.com/
107. http://www.womenchiropractors.com/
108. Hughes S and Bolton J. "Is chiropractic an effective treatment in infantile colic?" *Archives of Disease in Childhood.* (2002) 86: 382-384.
109. Jamison JR, Davies NJ. "Chiropractic Management of Cow's Milk Protein Intolerance in Infants With Sleep Dysfunction Syndrome: A Therapeutic Trial." *Journal of Manipulative and Physiological Therapeutics.* (2007, March) Vol. 30 (3): 247.
110. Jimenez S. "Supportive Pain Management Strategies." *Childbirth Education: Practice, Research, and Theory.* Nichols FH and Humenick SS eds. Saunders: Philadelphia, 1988.
111. Klaus M et al. "Maternal Assistance and Support in Labour: Father, Nurse, Midwife, or Doula?" *Clinical Obstetrics and Gynaecology.* (1992) Vol 4(4): 211-217.
112. Klebanoff MA, Carey JC et al. "Failure of Metronidazole to Prevent Preterm Delivery Among Pregnant Women with Asymptomatic *Trichomonas vaginalis* Infection." *The New England Journal of Medicine,* (2001, August 16) Vol 345: 487-493.
113. Kloss J. (1975). *Back to Eden: The Classical Guide to Herbal Medicine, Natural Foods and Home Remedies.* Woodbridge Press Publishing Co.: Santa Barbara, CA.
114. Klougart N, Nilsson N, et al. "Infantile colic treated by chiropractors: a prospective study of 316 cases." *Journal of Manipulative and Physiological Therapeutics.* (1989) 12: 281-288.
115. Koren G, Klinger G et al. "Fetal Pharmacotherapy." *Drugs.* (2002) Vol 62(5): 757-773.
116. Lazarou, Pomeranz et al. "Incidence of Adverse Drug Reactions in Hospitalized Patients." *Journal of the American Medical Association.* (1998, April) Vol 279(15): 1200.
117. Lerner B. "How Chiropractic Helps Newborns." www.mercola.com.
118. Levinson D. "Chiropractic Care and Exercise: A Winning Formula for a Healthy Pregnancy." *The American Chiropractor.* (1995) Vol 10-12, 39.
119. Li DK, Liu L et al. "Exposure to Non-Steroidal Anti-Inflammatory Drugs During Pregnancy and Risk of Miscarriage: Population Based Cohort Study." *British Medical Journal,* (2003, Aug. 16): 327-368.
120. Lieberman AB. (1992). *Easing Labour Pain.* Harvard Common Press; Boston, MA.
121. Martin SE. "New Baby Ergonomics: Tricks to Prevent the Aches and Strains That Come with the Territory." *Today's Parent Baby and Toddler.* (2004: Autumn/Winter).

122. McKeever TM, Lewis SA et al. "Antibiotic Use During Pregnancy Tied with Asthma Risk." *American Journal of Respiratory and Critical Care Medicine*. (2002, September 15) Vol 166(6): 827-832.

123. Mercer C, Nook BC. The efficacy of chiropractic spinal adjustments as a treatment protocol in the management of infantile colic. In: Haldeman S, Murphy B, eds. *Fifth Biennial Congress of the World Federation of Chiropractic*. Auckland, (1999) 170-171.

124. Miller J. (2005, November 15th). "Pediatric Essentials for the DC: From Principles to Practice." Lecture presented, Vancouver, BC.

125. Mitchell B, et al. "Attachments of the Ligamentum Nuchae to Cervical Posterior Spinal Dura and the Lateral Part of the Occipital Bone." *Journal of Manipulative and Physiological Therapeutics*. (1998, March/April) Vol 21(3).

126. Mohrbacher N. (2003). *Positioning Your Baby at the Breast*. La Leche League International: Publication No. 107, www.lllc.ca.

127. Mongan M. (2005). *HypnoBirthing®: The Mongan Method: A Natural Approach to a Safe, Easier, More Comfortable Birthing*. (3rd ed.). Health Communications Inc: Deerfield Beach, FL.

128. Moore TJ, Weiss SR, et al. "Reported Adverse Drug Events in Infants and Children Under Two Years of Age." *Pediatrics*. (2002:110) Vol 5: e53.

129. Moore CCCS. "All About Epidurals—Researching Your Options for Pain Relief." *www.iparenting.com*.

130. Mortensen E, Michaelsen K et al. "The Association Between Duration of Breastfeeding and Adult Intelligence." *Journal of the American Medical Association*. (2002) 287: 2365-2371.

131. Muhs G, Alderson S. "The Effects of Mild Compression on Spinal Nerve Roots With Implications for Models of Vertebral Subluxation and the Clinical Effects of Chiropractic Adjustment: A Review of the Literature." *Journal of Vertebral Subluxation Research*. (2001, September).

132. Odent M. (1992). *The Nature of Birth and Breastfeeding*. Bergin & Harvey: Westport CT.

133. Ohm J. (2000). "Webster Technique Defined." *International Chiropractic Paediatric Association Newsletter*.

134. Ohm J. "Chiropractic and Pregnancy: Greater Comfort and Safer Births." *International Chiropractic Paediatric Association Newsletter*. (2002, May-June).

135. Olafsdottir E, Forshei S et al. "Randomised controlled trial of infantile colic treated with chiropractic spinal manipulation." *Archives of Disease in Childhood*. (2001) 84: 138-141.

136. Oliveira AO, Fileto C, Melis, MS. "Effect of Strenuous Maternal Exercise Before and During Pregnancy on Rat Progeny Renal Function." *Brazilian Journal of Medical and Biological Research*. (2004) Vol 37: 907:911.

137. Olsen SF, Secher NJ. "Low Consumption of Seafood in Early Pregnancy as a Risk Factor for Preterm Delivery: Prospective Cohort Study." *British Medical Journal*, (2002) Vol 324: 447-450.

138. Penna M. "Pregnancy and Chiropractic Care." *American Chiropractic Association Journal of Chiropractic*. (1989) Vol 26: 31-33.

139. Perez P. (1997). *The Nurturing Touch at Birth*. Cutting Edge Press: Katy, TX.

140. Prescott JW. "Ten Principles of Mother-Infant Bonding for Health, Happiness and Harmony." *Institute of Humanistic Science*.

141. Province of British Columbia, Ministry for Children and Families. (1998). *Baby's Best Chance: Parent's Handbook of Pregnancy and Baby Care*. 5th ed. Macmillan Canada: Victoria, BC.

142. Province of British Columbia, Ministry of Health Planning and Ministry of Social Services. (2002). 1st ed. *Toddler's First Steps: A Best Chance Guide to Parenting Your Six-Month-to Three-Year-Old*. MacMillan Canada: Victoria, BC.

143. Pruiksma P. Pregnancy and Nutrition. Various Handouts.

144. Public Health Nutritionists in the Region of Peel Health Department. (2000). "Nutrition Matters—Pregnant or Breastfeeding? Get the Facts on Herbal Products and Teas." Toronto Public Health: Toronto, ON.

145. Rabe T. (1997). "Oh, Baby, the Places You'll Go!" Dr. Seuss Enterprises LP. Random House: Toronto, Canada.

146. Richards M, Hardy R et al. "Birth Weight and Cognitive Function in the British 1946 Cohort: Longitudinal Population Based Study." *British Medical Journal*. (2001) Vol 322: 199-203.

147. Sale R. "Looking into the Eyes of the Dragon—Transforming Pregnancy Fears." *Mothering Magazine*. (1999: September-October) 62-66.

148. Schaffer JI, Bloom SL et al. "A Randomized Trial of the Effects of Coached vs. Uncoached Maternal Pushing During the Second Stage of Labour on Postpartum Pelvic Floor Structure and Function." *American Journal of Obstetrics and Gynecology*. (2005, May) 192 (5): 1692-1696.

149. Shanley L. "Changing Fear/Tension/Pain into Faith/Relaxation/Pleasure" *www.unassistedchildbirth.com*.

150. Simkin P, Whalley J et al (1991). *Pregnancy, Childbirth, and the Newborn*. Meadowbrook Press: Deephaven, MN.

151. Simkin P. (1989) *The Birth Partner*. Harvard Common Press: Boston, MA.

152. Solter A. (1996). "What To Do When Your Baby Cries." *The Aware Baby*. Shining Star Press: Goleta, CA.

153. St. Leger AM. Pregnancy and Nutrition. Various Handouts.

154. St. Mary's Hospital Rehabilitation Services-Physiotherapy. "Post-Natal and Post-Caesarean Exercises." Handout.

155. St. Mary's Hospital Take Home Instructions. "Jaundice in Newborns." Handout.

156. Stengler M. (2001). *The Natural Physician's Healing Therapies.* Prentice Hall Press: Paramus, NJ.

157. Thomas P. "Aspartame and Phenylalanine May Alter Brain Growth in the Foetus." *Medical World News.* http://www.wnho.net/the_ecologist_aspartame_report.htm.

158. Troussier B, Davoine P et al. "Back Pain in School Children: A Study Among 1178 Pupils." *Scandinavian Journal of Rehabilitative Medicine.* (1994) 26:143-46.

159. Ursell A. (2001). *Vitamins and Mineral Handbook.* Dorling Kindersley Ltd: New York, NY.

160. US Environmental Protection Agency (2003, March 28). "Teflon Has Been Linked to Birth Defects and Infertility." *Environmental Working Group.*

161. US FDA Warning posted on Medscape Alert (07/20/2006) "SSRI Use in Pregnancy Linked to Risk for Pulmonary Hypertension in Newborns." http://www.fda.gov/medwatch.

162. Vallone S. "Chiropractic Evaluation and Treatment of Musculoskeletal Dysfunction in Infants Demonstrating Difficulty Breastfeeding." Journal of Clinical Chiropractic Pediatrics, (2004) Vol. 5: 1: 349-361.

163. Verny T, Kelly J. (1981). *The Secret Life of the Unborn Child: How You Can Prepare Your Baby for a Happy, Healthy Life.* Dell Publishing: New York, NY.

164. Verny T, Weintraub P. (1992). *Nurturing the Unborn Child.* Dell Publishing: New York, NY.

165. Villar J, Merialdi M et al. "Nutritional Interventions During Pregnancy for the Prevention or Treatment of Maternal Morbidity and Preterm Delivery: An Overview of Randomized Controlled Trials." *Journal of Nutrition.* (2003, May) Vol 133:1606S-1625S.

166. Walker N, O'Brien B. "The Relationship Between Method of Pain Management During Labour and Birth Outcomes." *Clinical Nursing Research.* (1999, May 8) Vol 2: 119-134.

167. Waller DK, Shaw GM et al. "Prepregnancy Obesity as a Risk Factor for Structural Birth Defects." *Arch Pediatr Adolesc Med.* (2007, August) Vol 161:745-750.

168. Wang SM, Dezinno P et al. "Low Back Pain During Pregnancy: Prevalence, Risk Factors and Outcomes." *Obstetrics and Gynaecology.* (2004, July) Vol 104(1): 65-70.

169. Weed S. (1986). *Wise Woman Herbal Childbearing Year.* Ash Tree: Woodstock, NY.

170. Wiberg JMM, Nordsteen J et al. "The short-term effect of spinal manipulation in the treatment of infantile colic: a randomised controlled

trial with a blinded observer." *Journal of Manipulative and Physiological Therapeutics.* (1999) 22: 517-522.

171. Wisborg K, Kesmodal U, et al. "Maternal Consumption of Coffee During Pregnancy and Stillbirth and Infant Death in the First Year of Life: Prospective Study." *British Medical Journal.* (2003) Vol 326: 420-423.

172. Zhang C, Williams MA, et al. "Vitamin C and the Risk of Pre-eclampsia—Results from Dietary Questionnaire and Plasma Assay." *Epidemiology,* (2002, July), 13: 409-416.

173. Zwelling E. "Get Moving! Exercise During Pregnancy." *www.pampers.com.*

Appendix One

Affirmations for Easy, Comfortable Birthing

- I am involved in a wonderful experience.
- I welcome this experience with such happiness.
- I am taking good care of myself for both my baby and myself.
- I am learning to relax more every day.
- I look forward to my baby's birth with such joy.
- I am a happy person; I am doing what I love to do.
- I put all fear aside as I prepare for the birth of my baby.
- All doubts are put aside as I look forward to my baby's birth.
- I am relaxed and happy that my baby is finally coming to me.
- I am focussed on a smooth, easy birth.
- I am creating a safe, healthy birth for my baby and myself.
- I am ready and able to have my baby now.
- I trust my body to know what it needs to do.
- My mind is relaxed; my body is relaxed.
- I am serene, calm, peaceful, and without stress.
- I feel confident; I feel safe; I feel secure.
- My muscles work in complete harmony to make birthing easier.
- I can labour in perfect harmony with nature.
- Childbirth is a normal, healthy event.
- I keep my mind calm and peaceful.
- I will be conscious and competent from the beginning of my birth experience to the end.
- I feel a natural anaesthesia flowing through my body.
- I relax as we move quickly and easily through each stage of birth.
- My cervix opens outward and allows my baby to ease down.
- I fully relax and turn my birthing over to nature.
- I see my baby coming smoothly from my womb.
- My baby's birth will be easy because I am so relaxed.

- I breathe correctly and eliminate tension.
- I feel my body gently swaying with relaxation.
- I turn my birthing over to my baby and my body.
- I am prepared for whatever happens during my birthing.
- My baby moves gently along its journey.
- Each contraction of my body brings my baby closer to me.
- The power of my uterine contractions will carry my baby from the womb.
- I deepen my relaxation as I move further into labour.
- I am totally relaxed and at ease.
- My body remains still and limp.
- I meet each contraction with only my breath; my body is at ease.
- I release my birthing over to my body and my baby.
- I bring myself into deeper relaxation.
- I slowly breathe up with each contraction, filling a balloon with my breath.
- I put all fear aside and welcome my baby with happiness and joy.
- I am ready and able to have my baby now.

[Adapted from *HypnoBirthing®: The Mongan Method: A Natural Approach to a Safe, Easier, More Comfortable Birthing*.]

Appendix Two

Rose Opening Visualization

"My cervix is opening like a blossoming rose, allowing my baby to emerge."

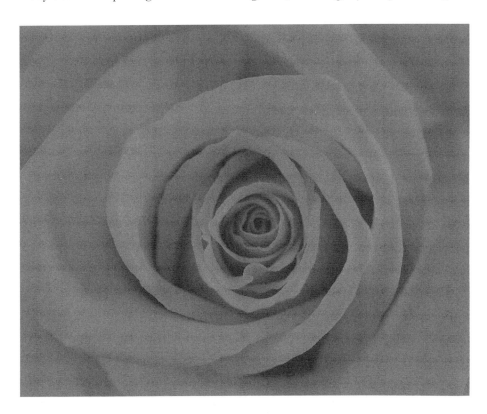

Appendix Three

A Plausible Cause of Infertility Discovered

Article by Barbara Sturm, DC

According to the Centers for Disease Control, more than six million women in the United States are infertile, and over nine million use some kind of infertility service.

A series of research papers regarding infertility published in the world-renowned *Journal Of Vertebral Subluxation Research* (www.jvsr.com) suggests that chiropractic adjustments, performed by chiropractors to address nerve interference caused by spinal distortions, could offer hope to many infertile women with their dreams of becoming mommies.

The twelve studies in the series found that chiropractic had positive results regardless of the woman's age, number of years infertile, previous medical intervention or health history including miscarriages, blocked fallopian tubes, amenorrhea, colitis, or trauma. This is truly remarkable news given the broad scope of possibilities for women from all walks and histories.

"Insult, Interference and Infertility: An Overview of Chiropractic Research," the first article of the series, reviewed fourteen retrospective articles on the possible effect of spinal problems on fertility. All of the women in these studies were found to have vertebral subluxations—misalignments and/or related problems of the spine that interfere with how the nerves work. These problems in the spine can be corrected by chiropractors with specific adjustments to the affected spinal area.

The stress histories of these infertile women included—but were not limited to—previous motor vehicle accidents, childhood falls, blocked fallopian tubes, scoliosis, and work stress that affected both mind and body. All of the women became pregnant after their subluxations were detected and corrected.

Vertebral subluxations rob countless people of an active, healthy, and fulfilling lifestyle. Infertility causes pain in the most sensitive of places—a woman's heart!

Appendix Four

Infant Formula Fortification Protocol

A mother's breast milk is nature's perfect and complete food for babies and can't even come close to being reproduced. With so many substances known to be present in breast milk that are unable to be replicated in breast milk substitutes (formula), plus all of the as-yet unidentified constituents, it should come as no great surprise that children today who are not breastfed are suffering from a vast myriad of illnesses and disorders.

The human brain is infinitely more sophisticated than the world's fastest computer, yet many people naively think that this wondrous organ can be perfectly constructed without any regard to the "raw materials" required. Building a properly functioning brain requires the right materials, just as building a computer would. Imagine trying to build a computer from scratch, without any microchips. Or trying to build a house without any lumber, bricks, steel, or other materials.

However, while there is no way to create a formula equal to breast milk, there are steps that can be taken to improve somewhat upon the standard formulas that are available.

One of the nutritional areas that is woefully inadequate in formulas is in regards to their fatty acid content. With all of the anti-fat propaganda going on these days, most people don't realize the critical importance of fat, especially with infants. Not only is the quantity important, but the quality and breakdown of the types of fat supplied as well. After all, the brain is sixty per cent lipid (fat). Of this fat, approximately twelve per cent is arachidonic acid (AA) and seventeen per cent is docosahexaenoic acid (DHA).

Many people have heard about the benefits and importance of the Omega-3 fatty acids DHA and EPA, found primarily in fish. The importance of DHA in the infant's diet recently prompted many countries to allow formula producers to fortify their products with DHA, as well as AA. Currently, DHA/AA enhanced formulas are available, although not mandatory, throughout most of Canada and Europe. Unfortunately, this small step still does not provide infants the nutrients they desperately require, due to several problems.

First of all, the DHA added to the formulas, obtained from microalgae, is highly oxidized. Additionally, DHA and AA are not the sole fat constituents of breast milk. Fortifying with them is a step in the right direction, but still leaves out plenty of important substances. In an effort to help people provide their infants with the best possible nutrition, we often instruct mothers to "create" fortified formulas. But of course we insist that mothers breastfeed if at all possible or even obtain fresh breast milk from a lactating friend or relative, if they have adopted a baby, or can't breastfeed for some reason. For the infant to remain as healthy as possible, he must obtain a proper balance of all the essential fats, which is difficult to impossible, especially when you are changing Mother Nature and trying to create a formula.

However, below is a basic formula fat fortification protocol, which attempts to come as close as possible to "the real thing":

> Cod liver oil—one cc/one millilitre per ten pounds of body weight
> Organic egg yolk—one yolk daily added at four months of age
> Organic cream ideally non-pasteurized and non-homogenized.
> Pure organic sesame, walnut, safflower, sunflower, oils (rotate with above)—one teaspoon/five millilitres daily
> One teaspoon/five millilitres high quality coconut oil. This oil needs to be heated to seventy-six degrees Fahrenheit (twenty-five degrees Celsius) to become a liquid.

Supplemental oils like fish oils can't be added to bottles because they will adhere to the sides, so it is necessary to administer directly into the mouth. But base oils as safflower, sunflower and sesame can be blended into the formula.

It is important, if not breastfeeding, to use one of the commercially available formulas as a "base" from which to fortify the infant's diet. Although some people might be tempted to create their own homemade formula, I don't recommend this approach, as it is just too dangerous that something could be inadvertently left out or added in too great a quantity. A mistake could cost an infant his life. Nutramagen or Alimentum can be used as a base infant formula and 'doctored up' with nutritional perks. Both of these formulas are acceptable in regard to the 'allergic' aspect, and are the ones usually used when children cannot tolerate anything. Of course, they are also the most expensive.

Fortified Commercial Formula

Makes about thirty-five ounces/1.1 litres
This stopgap formula can be used in emergencies, or when the ingredients for homemade formula are unavailable.
One cup/250 millilitres low-iron, milk-based powdered formula,
[Nutramigen or Alimentum are best and better tolerated but are more expensive]
29 ounces/900 millilitres boiled, filtered water
One large raw organic free-range egg yolk
[Do not give egg yolk to an infant unless older than four months of age]
One-teaspoon/five millilitres cod liver oil
Place all ingredients in a blender or food processor and blend thoroughly. Place 6-8 ounces in a very clean glass bottle. Store the rest in a very clean glass jar in the refrigerator for the next feedings. Attach a clean nipple to the bottle and set in a pan of simmering water until formula is warm but not hot to the touch, shake well and feed to baby.
[Never heat formula in a microwave oven as it destroys nutrients and may cause unsafe hot spots!]

If your baby is premature, one additional area of fortification is in the area of free amino acids, most notably taurine. This nutrient is also critical for infant development and is found in human milk but not in cow's milk. Although many formulas add some taurine, it has been shown that formula-fed infants have lower levels of taurine in their blood than breastfed infants do, even when the formula has added taurine.

Contrary to the advice given by some, soy milk, rice milk, almond milk, or carrot juice, even if organic and homemade, are most definitely not acceptable substitutes for breast milk, or even for formula.

For those mothers who are breastfeeding, it is important to realize that the essential fatty acid content of her breast milk coincides with what she eats. Therefore, her diet is very important for the health of her baby. One of the most important things that a breastfeeding mother can do is to avoid foods containing trans fats, such as margarine and anything with hydrogenated or partially hydrogenated oils. While one can't guarantee that taking the steps outlined above will completely eliminate problems such as ADD/ADHD and other behavioural problems, developmental problems, autism, visual difficulties, and others, I believe that it is a strong possibility that it could help to reduce their incidence, although it is important to always remember that BREAST IS BEST.

PLEASE recognize that soy formula is an unmitigated disaster for infants and should never be used. It is high in:

◊   manganese
◊   aluminum
◊   phytoestrogens that will harm your baby

For more information on soy formula, please check out: www.mercola.com.

Alternatively a raw milk formula can be made:

Milk-Based Formula

Makes thirty-six ounces/1.2 litres
This milk-based formula takes account of the fact that human milk is richer in whey, lactose, vitamin C, niacin, and long-chain polyunsaturated fatty acids compared to cow's milk but leaner in casein (milk protein).
Use only truly expeller-expressed oils in the formula recipes, otherwise they may lack vitamin E.
The ideal milk for baby, if he cannot be breastfed, is clean, whole raw milk from goats. If goats are not available, then milk from cows certified free of disease, that feed on green grass pasture would be a second best choice.
For sources of good quality milk, see: **www.realmilk.com**
If the only choice available to you is commercial milk, choose whole milk, preferably organic and unhomogenized, and culture it with a piima or **Kefir Culture** to restore enzymes.
Two cups/500 millilitres whole milk, raw (non-pasteurized) milk from pasture-fed cows
One-quarter cup/seventy-five millilitres liquid whey
Four tablespoons/sixty millilitres lactose
One-teaspoon/five millilitres bifidobacterium infantis
Two or more tablespoons/thirty millilitres good quality raw cream (non-pasteurized),
[more if you are using milk from Holstein cows]
One-teaspoon/five millilitres **cod liver oil**
One-teaspoon/five millilitres expeller-expressed organic sunflower oil
One-teaspoon/five millilitres extra virgin organic olive oil

Two-teaspoons/ten millilitres coconut oil
Two-teaspoons/ten millilitres nutritional yeast flakes
Two-teaspoons/ten millilitres gelatin
One and seven-eighths $(1+\frac{7}{8})$ of a cup/475 millilitres filtered water
One-quarter teaspoon/one millilitre acerola powder
Add gelatin to water and heat gently until gelatin is dissolved. Place
all ingredients in a very clean glass or stainless steel container and mix
well. To serve, pour six to eight ounces into a very clean glass bottle,
attach nipple and set in a pan of simmering water. Heat until warm but
not hot to the touch, shake bottle well and feed baby.
[Never, never heat formula in a microwave oven!]

Note: If you are using the Lact-Aid, mix all ingredients well in a blender.

Goat's Milk Formula

Although goat's milk is rich in fat, it must be used with caution in infant feeding as it lacks folic acid and is low in vitamin B12, both of which are essential to the growth and development of the infant. Inclusion of nutritional yeast to provide folic acid is essential. To compensate for low levels of vitamin B12, add two teaspoons frozen organic raw chicken liver, finely grated to the batch of formula. Be sure to begin egg yolk feeding at four months.

[Adapted from: www.mercola.com]

Index

C

latch 84, 85, 88, 89, 122 *see also breastfeeding*

laxative 50, 86 *see also elimination, constipation*

leafy green vegetables 73

leg and foot cramps 49, 75, 76, 101

leg extension 83

leg inversions 74

lemon balm 77, 78, 81, 87

licorice root 55 *see herbs to use with caution during pregnancy*

lifting 32, 107, 116

lily of the valley 56 *see herbs to avoid during pregnancy*

linden flower 87

liver 14, 44, 50, 54, 77, 78, 101, 117, 145, 146, 147, 148

low spirits 50, 78 *see also depression*

lumbar roll 114

lying position 117 *see also sleeping*

M

mackerel 39, 43, 46

magnesium 45, 46, 47, 50, 78

manganese 45, 147

mango 77

marigold 56 *see herbs to avoid during pregnancy*

marshmallow root 52

massage 26, 27, 32, 70, 72, 73, 74, 75, 81, 84, 130, 132

mastitis 67, 68

ma huang 56 *see herbs to avoid during pregnancy*

Medicago sativa *see alfalfa*

meditation 78, 79, 80

menstrual troubles 50, 52, 101, 103

mental fogginess 79

mercury 39, 43, 46, 57, 73, 97 *see also heavy metals*

microwave 40, 146, 148

milk 20, 36, 43, 46, 49, 50, 56, 66, 67, 68, 77, 84, 85, 86, 87, 88, 90, 91, 92, 93, 122, 133, 144, 145, 146, 147

minerals 36, 40, 48, 49, 50

mint 45, 47, 76, 77, 78, 87

miscarriage 39, 41, 49, 52, 56, 61, 62, 65, 72, 77, 133, 142

mommy brain 79

mormon tea 56 *see herbs to avoid during pregnancy*

morning sickness 46, 49, 76

morphine 63, 82 *see also narcotics, opiates*

motherwort 55, 56, 78 *see herbs to use with caution during pregnancy*

motor vehicle accidents 65, 97, 142

moulding 88, 93

mountain daisy see Arnica Montana

mucus in the baby's lungs 67, 91

mugwort 56 *see herbs to avoid during pregnancy*

mullein 74

muscle spasm(s) 49, 52, 70 *see also cramps*

musculoskeletal 92, 130, 131, 136

N

narcotics 20, 30

nasal stuffiness 73

natural childbirth 19, 20, 21, 124, 132

nausea 58, 59, 60, 61, 62, 64, 76, 77 *see also morning sickness*

neck pain 101, 125

nerve(s) 14, 45, 51, 45, 66, 75, 86, 88, 90, 95, 96, 97, 98, 99, 101, 103, 104, 122, 123, 124, 125, 126, 134, 142

nerve interference 126, 142

nervous system 14, 38, 51, 64, 94, 96, 97, 98, 99, 100, 101, 103, 111, 124, 125

nettle leaves (Urtica dioica) 45, 47, 49, 50, 53, 70, 73, 77, 88

newborn 20, 38, 88, 92, 93, 124, 126, 129, 133, 135, 136

progressive relaxation 80

prolonged labour 80, 92, 111

protein 36, 39, 43, 45, 46, 73, 76, 85, 91, 92, 108, 133, 147

Pulsatilla 59, 60, 61, 62, 64, 66, 67

R

ragweed 56 *see herbs to avoid during pregnancy*

rash 91

recurrent ear infections 126

red clover 47, 49

red raspberry leaf (Rubus idaeus) 45, 47, 49, 50, 53, 56, 77, 79, 81, 86, 87, 88

regional analgesia 30 *see epidural(s)*

regurgitating 91 *see also gastro-esophageal reflux, heartburn*

Relaxin 104, 120

reptiles 39

retracing 100

returning the uterus, perineum and abdominal muscles to normal more quickly 81

rice milk 146

rocking 30, 32, 71, 90

rose hip 87

round ligament pain 72

Rubus idaeus *see red raspberry leaf*

rue 56 *see herbs to avoid during pregnancy*

S

sacroiliac 101, 104, 125

safety belt(s) 114

safe sex 42

safflower oil 77, 145

saffron 56 *see herbs to avoid during pregnancy*

salt 44, 45, 46, 73, 75, 78, 86

sardines 43, 46

sassafras root 56 *see herbs to avoid during pregnancy*

sauna 41, 71

sciatica 101

scoliosis 125, 143

scothbroom 56 *see herbs to avoid during pregnancy*

seat belt(s) *see safety belt(s)*

seizures 91

senna leaves 56 *see herbs to avoid during pregnancy*

Sepia 58, 60, 61, 64, 65

sesame 45, 46, 145

sexually transmitted diseases 37

shark 39, 43

shellfish 43, 45

Silica 68, 69

silica 45, 47

simethicone 90

singing 90

sitting 32, 59, 74, 82, 101, 113, 114, 123

sitz bath 54, 74, 81

skullcap 78

sleep(ing) 51, 61, 65, 70, 82, 87, 89, 90, 92, 97, 99, 107, 116, 117, 120, 130, 133

slings *see front carriers*

slippery elm (Ulmus fulva) 51, 52, 77

slowing down of the digestive tract 76 *see also elimination, constipation*

smoke, smoking 37, 90, 107, 108, 131

sore nipples 67, 84, 88 *see also nipples*

sore throat 61, 101

soy 92, 146, 147

spearmint 77, 78

spinach 44, 45, 73

spinal decay 97, 98

spinal dysfunction 96, 97 *see also subluxation*

spine 14, 40, 71, 94, 96, 97, 98, 99, 101, 103, 104, 107, 110, 111, 113, 116, 117, 121, 122, 123, 124, 125, 126, 142